Shaping the Breast

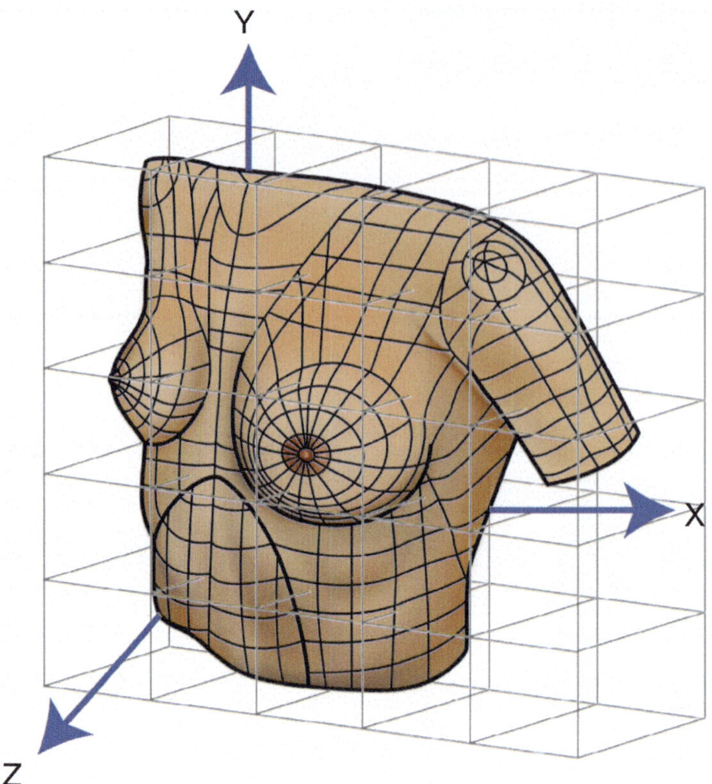

Y
X
Z

Kiya Movassaghi
Editor

Shaping the Breast

A Comprehensive Approach in Augmentation, Revision, and Reconstruction

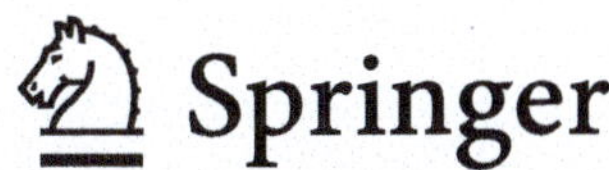

Editor
Kiya Movassaghi, MD, DMD, FACS
Plastic Surgery
Oregon Health & Science University
Portland, OR
USA

ISBN 978-3-030-59779-5 ISBN 978-3-030-59777-1 (eBook)
https://doi.org/10.1007/978-3-030-59777-1

This Springer imprint is published by the registered company Springer Nature Switzerland AG
The registered company address is: Gewerbestrasse 11, 6330 Cham, Switzerland

To my father, Amir-Houshang Movassaghi, MD, whose kindness and caring energy for others and passion for medicine forged the way for me. His dedication to fulfilling one's potential was a constant source of inspiration. His mantra was, "When you love your job you don't work," and it has always resonated with me.

To my two sons, Nima and Aria, who I love dearly. They give me so much joy and have helped me become a better person.

To my best friend and wife, Niloo. She has been my constant companion, providing wisdom, strength, comfort, support, and loyalty. Her endless and unconditional love flows effortlessly, and she enriches the lives of everyone that she meets. At times this book took me away from my family, but despite late nights, someone was always waiting to greet me when I came home.

To my patients, who have entrusted me with the sacred opportunity to help them as their surgeon. It has been truly an honor to be part of their surgical journey.

Kiya Movassaghi

Preface

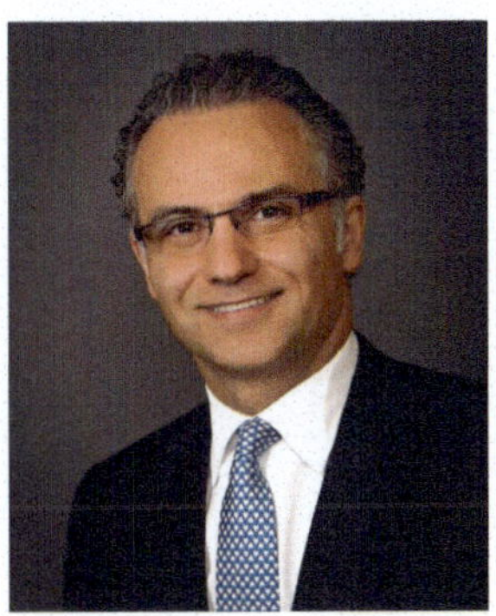

Shaping the Breast grew out of my discontent as a resident and later as a practicing surgeon with the lack of a precise roadmap to approach the fundamentals of breast surgery to achieve optimal results. Despite the vast number of publications on breast surgery, I felt that there was a deficit in easy-to-process yet detailed source of information that brought all of the concepts together. With observation, surgical experience, and better devices, my approach to breast surgery has evolved from "volumizing" the breast to "shaping" the breast. This vision was the launching pad for the book.

Chapter 1 is an extensive, in-depth, and detailed presentation of best practices in breast surgery. It introduces the readers to the process of successful breast surgery, which includes patient interview, physical analysis, biodimensional planning, surgical marking and execution, and postoperative care. Chapter 2 builds on the principles learned in Chap. 1 and covers augmentation mastopexy, which is one of the most challenging situations in aesthetic breast surgery. Chapter 3 is about the evolving role of fat injection in breast surgery, with an emphasis on composite breast augmentation. It provides readers with the realistic expectations that can be achieved by this procedure, something that is not always fully disclosed. Chapter 4 discusses the expanding field of breast reconstruction, covering both alloplastic and autologous breast reconstruction with good references to build on. Lastly, Chap. 5 brings together all the principles learned in the first four chapters and applies them to the management of very challenging but commonly seen breast cases. In addition, some technical pearls are introduced in this chapter.

While no single textbook can provide an encyclopedic presentation of such a broad-based discipline, this book has been designed to provide a foundation of information useful at every level of experience and to stimulate further self-directed education. The authors have been selected to provide information based on their experience, enthusiasm, and teaching skills. You will recognize many as the current leaders in their fields. It has been my privilege to work with this dedicated group of educators and surgeons, and I hope that the women in your care will benefit from their efforts.

Portland, OR, USA Kiya Movassaghi

Acknowledgments

I have been fortunate to learn from some of the best in plastic surgery at the Harvard Combined Plastic Surgery Program. They taught me critical thinking skills and always encouraged me to push the boundaries of plastic surgery. In particular, I would like to acknowledge the late Joseph Murphy, MD, the late Francis Wolfort, MD, the late Robert Goldwyn, MD, James May, MD, Michael Yaremchuk, MD, Elof Eriksson, MD, Joseph Upton MD, Julian Pribaz, MD, and John Mulliken, MD. I also had the opportunity to train and learn from some of the legendary maxillofacial surgeons at Massachusetts General Hospital, in particular the late Walter Guralnick, DMD, Bruce Donoff, DMD, MD, and Leonard Kaban, DMD, MD.

In addition, the foundation for this book came to fruition after my two visits to Charles Randquist, MD, in Stockholm, Sweden. He is not only a visionary in the field of breast surgery but he is also incredibly gracious.

Lastly, a word of gratitude for my aesthetic fellows, who bring energy, excitement, and new ideas to my world and who along the way have helped me sharpen my skills and instincts.

Kiya Movassaghi

Contents

Contributors

Louis P. Bucky, MD Bucky Plastic Surgery, Ardmore, PA, USA

M. Bradley Calobrace, MD, FACS CaloAesthetics Plastic Surgery Center, Louisville, KY, USA

University of Louisville Division of Plastic Surgery, Louisville, KY, USA

University of Kentucky Division of Plastic Surgery, Louisville, KY, USA

Jenna Cusic, MD Aesthetic Surgery Fellow, Movassaghi Plastic Surgery, Eugene, OR, USA

Chet Mays, MD CaloAesthetics Plastic Surgery Center, Louisville, KY, USA

University of Louisville Division of Plastic Surgery, Louisville, KY, USA

Kiya Movassaghi, MD, DMD, FACS Clinical Assistant Professor of Plastic Surgery, Oregon Health & Science University, Portland, OR, USA

Movassaghi Plastic Surgery & Ziba Medical Spa, Eugene, OR, USA

ASAPS Endorsed Aesthetic Fellowship, Eugene, OR, USA

Maurice Y. Nahabedian, MD Department of Plastic Surgery, Virginia Commonwealth University – Inova Branch, McLean, VA, USA

Kevin J. Shultz, MD Upstate Plastic Surgery, Greer, SC, USA

James M. Smartt Jr, MD Bucky Plastic Surgery, Ardmore, PA, USA

1 Shaping the Breast: Optimizing Outcomes in Breast Augmentation

Kiya Movassaghi and Jenna Cusic

Introduction

Breast augmentation and breast reconstruction are frequent indications for the use of breast implants. With time, heightened patient and surgeon expectations have evolved along with improvements in implant technology and surgical technique. Breast augmentation surgery continues to be one of the most frequently performed aesthetic surgeries around the world with over 300,000 cases per year performed in the United States alone [1].

These trends in breast reconstruction and augmentation have equated to a rise in the number of revisionary surgeries, which can be as high as 30–40% [2–4]. The most common reasons for revision surgery include capsular contracture, implant malposition, asymmetry, implant rupture, desire for size change, ptosis, wrinkling/rippling, or hematoma/seroma [4, 5]. In order for breast augmentation and reconstruction practice to advance and improve, the surgeons must constantly strive toward fewer complications and reoperations, predictable long-term results, and a better experience for the patient. The surgeon must be attentive in the communication with the patient and adhere to certain principles, both during implant selection and surgery. As with any craft, the improved outcome can only be achieved by adhering to the fundamentals, which will be the focus of this chapter. There are three determinants of a successful implant-based breast surgery: patient factors, implant factors, and surgical factors.

Patient Factors

Like any other surgery, the process starts with the initial consultation. During the consultation, it is imperative to evaluate several factors that are related to both the patient's state of mind and body characteristics. Central to the process of selecting patients for any type of aesthetic surgical procedure is the well-being and safety of the patient. The surgeon and staff must be able to differentiate between patients who are impulsive and not emotionally stable and those that are stable and informed. Furthermore, patients under age 18 cannot consult without an accompanying parent. Keep in mind that breast augmentation may be performed with saline implants in patients aged 18 and older and with silicone implants in patients aged 22 and older [6]. Breast reconstruction

K. Movassaghi (✉)
Clinical Assistant Professor of Plastic Surgery, Oregon Health & Science University, Portland, OR, USA

Movassaghi Plastic Surgery & Ziba Medical Spa, Eugene, OR, USA

ASAPS Endorsed Aesthetic Fellowship, Eugene, OR, USA
e-mail: kiya@drmovassaghi.com

J. Cusic
Aesthetic Surgery Fellow, Movassaghi Plastic Surgery, Eugene, OR, USA

K. Movassaghi (ed.), *Shaping the Breast*, https://doi.org/10.1007/978-3-030-59777-1_1

with either saline or silicone implants may be performed at any age [6].

Correctly selecting patients is difficult. It requires verbal communication skills, genuine interest in the patients, and the ability to listen. While some of these capabilities can be learned through academic studies, a successful patient selection also requires a great deal of experience. For the young plastic surgeon, it is therefore very important to have the proper mentor. Wrongly scheduling a patient for surgery will be detrimental to the patient, the surgeon, and the surgical practice. At times, the best surgery is the one never performed [7].

Medical History

In the authors' practice, the patient's physical health is carefully evaluated by the surgeon and the anesthesiologist. Surgery can be scheduled if the medical risk of the procedure is expected to be negligible. Furthermore, if the patient has an ongoing psychiatric condition, she should have documentation from her treating doctor, stating that she is suitable for surgery and that the procedure would not worsen her condition [7].

Patient Motivation

During the consultation, the patient should seem comfortable with her decision and not be hesitant. It is imperative to ascertain that it is the firm will of the patient herself to follow through with a breast augmentation. It should not be a spur of the moment decision, and the patient should have spent significant time evaluating the procedure and its associated risks. Furthermore, even though many patients will relay that they have been considering the procedure for as long as they can remember, the standard questions should always be "…and how come you have decided on this procedure right now?"

Importantly, the authors always assure that the patient is in a stable social situation and that she, for example, has not recently experienced an emotional trauma such as a divorce.

Body Dysmorphic Disorder

As when dealing with any cosmetic surgical procedure, it is important to exclude patients suffering from body dysmorphic disorder, as surgery only reinforces the condition. During the consultation it often becomes evident if a patient is suffering from body dysmorphic disorder or not, but at times a few screening questions are required. If the patient has a history of bulimia or anorexia, she should be declared healthy at least 6 months prior to the consultation [8, 9].

Body Characteristics

The characteristics of the patient's chest wall, existing breasts, and history of previous breast surgeries greatly influence the end result. Understanding the differences in anatomy and choosing the correct implants is imperative.

During recent decades, the range of implants on the market has increased steadily. Several implant systems from different manufacturers are now available with different fill ratio, profile (low, moderate, high, ultrahigh), gel cohesivity ("gummy, gummier and gummiest"), shape variation (teardrop vs. round) with flexibility in height, width, projection, and surface variations (smooth, microtexture, and macrotexture). With careful considerations, one can find a suitable implant that matches the patient's desire and anatomy. The sheer number of available implants might at first seem daunting, but as the chest wall shape and breast size among females in a uniform population usually do not vary greatly, a relatively small number of implants is required to solve most of the cases. In the authors' experience, a majority of breast augmentations can be performed using a select number of available implants. Furthermore, given the great implant diversity, it is possible to find and fit an implant for virtually every patient's features and desires. This enables fine-tuning and correction of even the most severe asymmetries and serves as a tool in a surgeon's constant strive toward perfection [10, 11].

Patient Expectations and Requests

The reason for which the patient is seeking breast implant surgery must be heard in the patient's own words. It is, however, imperative that the surgeon clarifies certain descriptive terms by the patient. For instance, many times when the patient indicates a desire for more "natural result," they may not mean a tear-shaped implant rather a soft but round upper pole. Similarly, many times when the patient request a "lift," they mean upper pole fullness and even a higher footprint. Often, a picture of the desired result that she finds appealing is helpful in determining her true wish.

Although it is ultimately the woman's choice for a certain volume, shape, and material for the implant, it is always the surgeon's responsibility to inform the patient which resulting shape is achievable given her specific body characteristics. Involving a patient in the implant selection process without risking long-term adverse consequences is a delicate balance. At times, patients present unrealistic expectations that make them unsuitable for surgery. An example is the very thin patient with ptotic breasts in need of a submuscular breast augmentation but who refuses a necessary mastopexy. Another example is the patient desiring very large implants that might look disproportionate and, more importantly, exert excessive pressure on the tissue. The surgeon together with the patient should choose implants based on the patient's chest wall and existing breast tissue in accordance with her desired final shape and volume. If after going through this process, the desired implant by the patient is unreasonable, the patient should be denied surgery [12, 13]. The surgeon must remind the patient that at times short-term satisfaction does not equate long-term durability when it comes to implant selection.

Much less frequent is the case with a patient who firmly requests extremely small implants. Implants that are too small or have the wrong shape could also lead to an unsatisfactory aesthetic result.

Patient Information and Education

Whether patients request too small or too large of implants is of course a highly subjective opinion. However, in order for us to strive for maximal satisfaction combined with less complication and reoperation rate, we need to educate the patients on the importance of the distribution of the volume as opposed to the absolute amount of volume. She needs to be educated that the "cc" is not as important as the distribution of the "cc." For example, a 200 cc highly cohesive round implant, 200 cc less cohesive round implant, or 200 cc tear-shaped implant will have different appearances in a thin patient, particularly in the upper pole, as well as the nipple projection (Figs. 1.1 and 1.2).

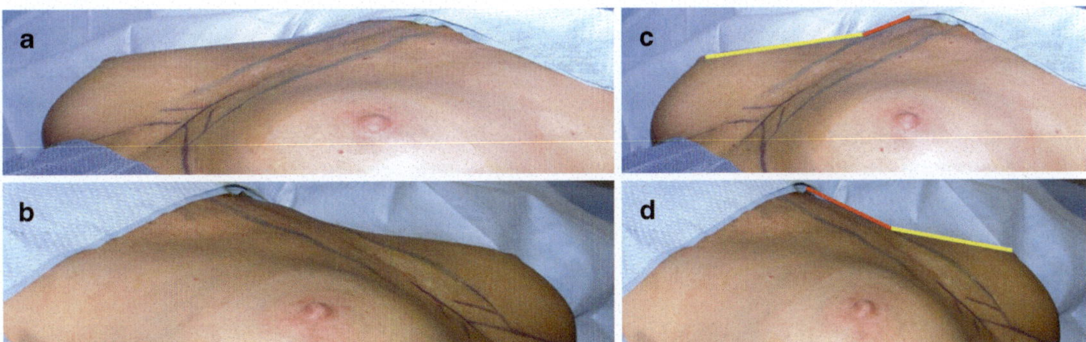

Fig. 1.1 Breast augmentation in the submuscular pockets with the same volume but different shape implants. A tall height tear-shaped implant with $Y > X$ is used on the right (**a**) and a round implant with $X = Y$ is used on the left (**b**). Note the difference in the volume of distribution in the upper pole between the two breasts with different shape but the same volume implants (**c**, **d**)

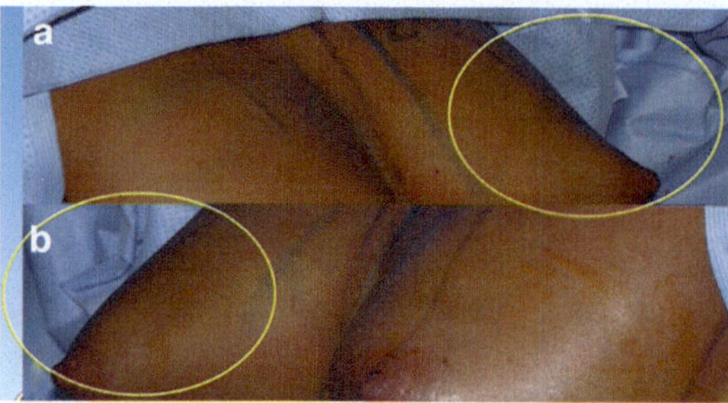

Fig. 1.2 Breast augmentation in the submuscular pockets with the same volume but different shape implants. A low-profile, tall height tear-shaped implant with $Y > X$ is used on the left (**a**) and a high-profile, round implant with $X = Y$ is used on the right (**b**). Note the difference in the upper pole volume of distribution

The education of the patient is of utmost importance in the preoperative phase. This transfer of information can be done via the website and through the consultation process. Computer analysis where the patient and surgeon review the patient's photos and analyze her anatomical features as they relate to the surgical plan provides a great opportunity to ensure that the patient fully understands what the surgeon sees and has planned (Fig. 1.3). These images will be saved as part of patient's record.

As part of the informed consent process, the patient must be made aware of all issues with implants such as capsular contracture, rippling/visibility, rupture, malposition, breast-implant-associated anaplastic large cell lymphoma (BIA-ALCL), especially with textured implants and the possibility of "breast implant illness" (BII) with all implants [14–17]. It is imperative that the patient understands that additional surgery might be required at some point in the future, and the implants are not permanent devices. The FDA recommends screening for detecting silicone breast implant rupture with an MRI or high resolution ultrasound 6 years after implants are placed and every 2-3 years thereafter [18]. This recommendation was based on data showing rupture rates are higher at 5–6 years after implantation, and knowledge that compliance with MRI with previous recommendations is poor [19].

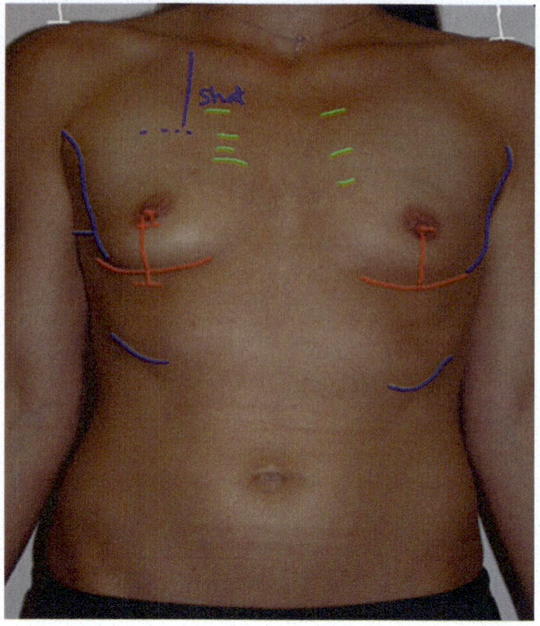

Fig. 1.3 A typical preoperative visit with the patient involves computer analysis discussing and documenting the patient's unique anatomical features and their potential influence on her outcome. This patient has scoliosis with uneven shoulders, high breast foot print, paucity of subcutaneous fat with visible ribs, uneven nipples, IMFs, and costal margins

Implant Factors

This is the most important influencer in a successful implant-based breast surgery. The notion that "all implants are created equal" is not true. The surface, the shell, the content, and the shape of the implants matter greatly, and one must understand the indications, the limitations, and alternatives for each device in order to achieve the optimal outcome. Evaluation of implants covers two areas: safety (toxicity, immunogenicity, teratogenicity, carcinogenicity) and efficacy (capsular contracture, deflation, palpability and rippling, pocket stability). The distinction between smooth and textured devices is of both efficacy and safety (BIA-ALCL). But why consider different implants for different situations? It is well known that implants with healthy soft tissue coverage behave well regardless of the type of implant but what about certain difficult situations such as the ptotic breast with thin and stretched out glandular tissue, the very thin patient, recurrent implant malposition, the tuberous/constricted breast, or breast reconstruction? These types of cases may benefit from a more advanced planning and implant selection.

Pocket Control

In order to have a successful and durable outcome, one must have pocket control which is influenced by friction (stability) and Newton's third law (in essence: controlled tissue expansion). The concept of friction is paramount in understanding implant stability. The greater the friction between the implant and surrounding tissue, the more stable the implant will be [20, 21]. Friction is defined by the following formula:

$$\text{Friction} = \mu(N)$$

where μ is the coefficient of friction, and N is the force pressing two objects together. μ is directly related to the materials used (all textured implants have higher μ compared to smooth implants), and N is directly related to fill ratio, implant cohesivity, and precise implant pocket creation; the more cohesive and higher fill ratio and tighter pockets having a larger N.

Newton's third law states that for every action there is a reaction. This is the guiding principle behind *controlled tissue expansion* (Fig. 1.4).

The more cohesive and textured implants give away less when pressed by the surrounding tissue, therefore have a stronger action–reaction. This results in a more controlled tissue expansion. In contrast, the less cohesive and underfilled smooth implants have weaker action–reaction with the surrounding tissue, which results in uncontrolled tissue expansion. The smooth round/non-cohesive implants will give over time because of gravity inferiorly (while standing) and laterally (while supine) resulting in uncontrolled tissue expansion. On the other hand, textured/highly cohesive gel implants (round or anatomic) will give the least, resulting in controlled expansion [22]. There are several patient and implant factors that are associated with less lower pole stretching and less uncontrolled tissue expansion. These include textured implants, cohesive implants, higher fill ratio implants, silicone implants, smaller and lower profile implants, and tight breast skin.

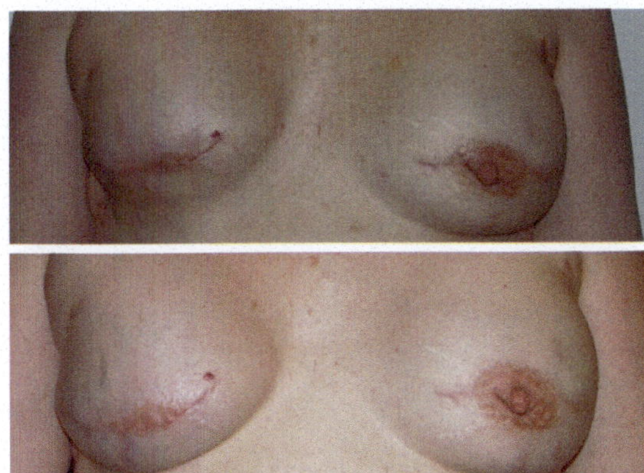

Fig. 1.4 This patient underwent bilateral mastectomies with skin sparing on the right and nipple sparing on the left with immediate stage I reconstruction with textured tissue expanders. The top photo is taken at the end of the expansion process, and the bottom photo is taken 4 months later before stage II. Note the controlled tissue expansion of the lower pole that has taken place with the textured devices on both sides, especially the right side

Physical Exam

Patient's torso is evaluated both anteriorly and posteriorly. Outside of the breast exam and measurements, the chest wall shape is important to note as some of the features may influence the implant selection. The shoulder levels and the presence of scoliosis, the curvature of the ribs (convex or concave), the curvature of axillary folds and tails, sternal shape, and visibility of the ribs are all assessed and documented. Scoliosis may contribute to the asymmetries of IMFs, nipple locations, and axillary silhouette. Scoliosis can cause vertical breast asymmetry requiring thoughtful implant positioning to minimize it. Similarly, the spinal rotation may contribute to the convexity or concavity of the ribs, and hence the fullness or flatness of the upper poles of the breasts and the projection of the breasts. The sternal shape variations with the pectus excavatum and carinatum (pigeon-shaped) chest representing the two ends of the spectrum require some adjustments in implant selection. Certain shapes make implant malposition more likely. A round thorax shape makes the breast axes diverge, causing the breasts to appear farther apart following augmentation and encourages lateral malposition, especially in the subpectoral pocket due to the lateral slope and the unfavorable lateral force of the pectoralis muscle. Similarly, the pectus excavatum shape encourages medial malposition due to the medial slope. A rectangular thorax makes the axes parallel, so that the breasts appear closer together postoperatively. Hemithorax asymmetry due to differences in shape or relative protrusion can create an uneven breast foundation, suggesting different size implants despite equivalent breast volumes (Fig. 1.5).

The height of the upper chest measured from mid clavicle to the top of the breast (CL:BR) may influence the vertical height of the implant that the patient can tolerate. Finally, the foot print of the breasts on the chest wall must be assessed: low, medium, or high (Fig. 1.6) [23].

Next, the breast measurements are done. These should include the true base width (TBW) and the existing base width (EBW), nipple to inframammary fold distance measured relaxed and under maximum stretch (N:IMF), areolar

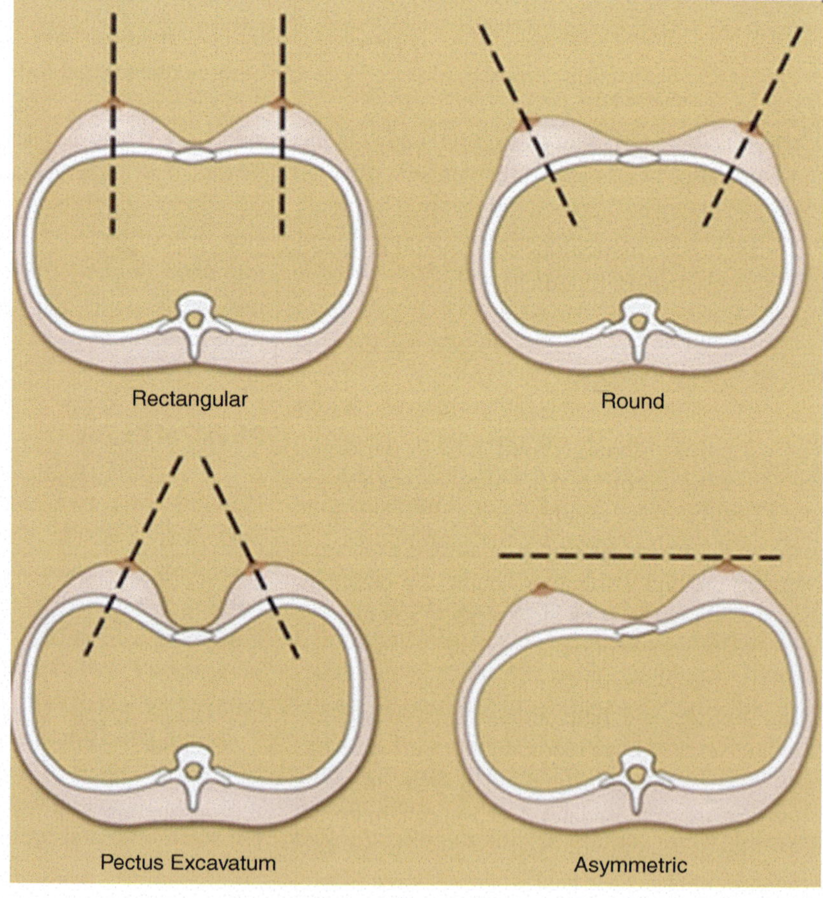

Fig. 1.5 The chest wall anatomy influences the platform upon which the implant sits. This can influence asymmetries, nipple axis, and potentiate certain implant malposition. (Used with permission of Wolters Kluwer Health, Inc., from Rehnke et al. [35])

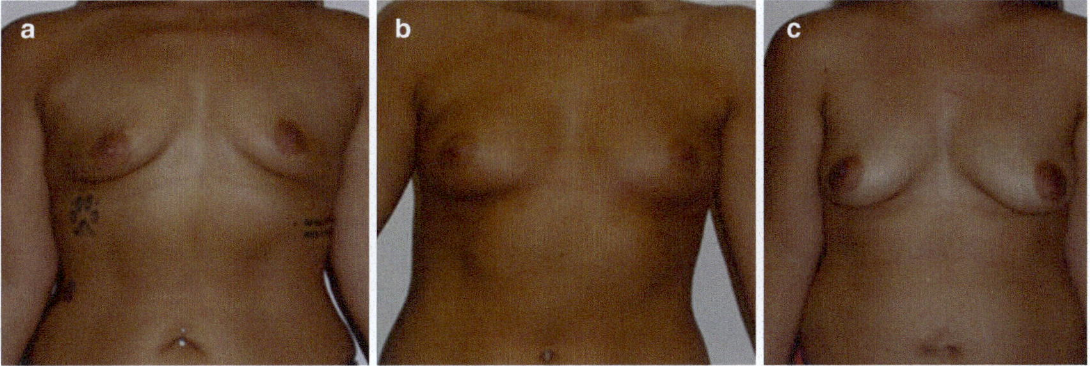

Fig. 1.6 The breasts can have a high (**a**), medium (**b**), and low (**c**) footprint. This greatly influences the implant chosen and the final outcome

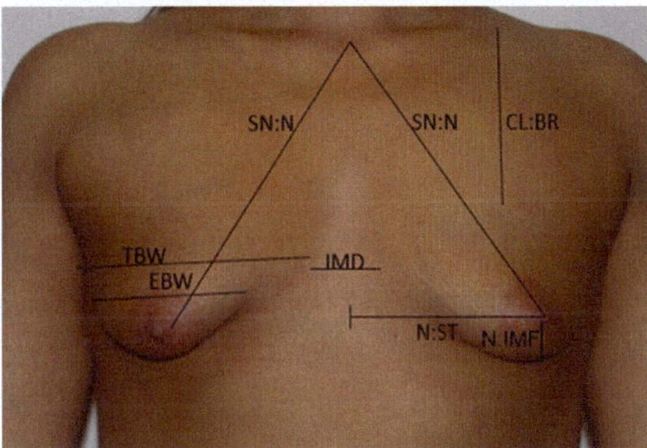

Fig. 1.7 Breast measurements

diameters (AD, transverse, and vertical), sternal notch to nipple distance (SN:N), nipple to mid sternum distance (N:ST), pinch test of the breast tissue laterally and medially and superiorly, nipple stretch test, and vertical excess in cases of ptosis [24–26] (Figs. 1.7 and 1.8).

Implant Selection

Once the patient exam is completed, the implant selection process is done [27, 28]. The implant selection process involves the surgeon's understanding of the patient's expectations and a careful assessment of the patient's chest wall and breasts. In order to understand what the patient is looking for, the surgeon must be attentive and may pose standard questions such as "describe the ideal shape of your breast." Often patients confuse the overall size and the volume of distribution. They may say: "I don't want to be too big" or "I want to still look natural" but want a more "fuller and round" upper pole when they are probed further. We sometimes find it helpful if the patients bring photos of breasts that they like.

The consultation should preferably take place in a peaceful environment, in front of a mirror where the patient is given the opportunity to express her desires. The considerations are then given to the implant dimensions and shape, implant surface, implant content, cohesivity, and fill ratio. Like any other three-dimensional structures, the implants have three dimensions of X, Y, and Z with the X being the width, Y being the height, and Z being the projection. The X is the most important and least negotiable dimension during implant selection as it is dictated by the true breast width (TBW) and the thickness of the breast tissue. By choosing an implant that is not too wide, the risk of future problems such as rippling, implant visibility, bottoming out or skin stretch is minimized. The X is determined by the following formula

$$X = \text{TBW} - \text{Thickness of breast tissue}$$

$$\text{Thickness of breast tissue} = \frac{1}{2}(\text{Medial pinch thickness} + \text{Lateral pinch thickness})$$

The SN-N and CL-BR distances, as well as upper chest anatomy and projection and patient desire for certain amount of fullness in the upper pole, provide directions on which Y the implant should have. Obviously, with a round implant, the X and Y are the same. Therefore, in the setting of a short upper chest or high foot print, one must be careful to avoid too wide or too cohesive of an implant. In this case, an appropriately selected X will result into a relatively too tall of Y if a round implant ($X = Y$) is chosen. Alternatively, one can select a tear-shaped implant with a shorter Y than X to address the short upper chest (Figs. 1.9 and 1.10).

Finally, the Z is the most negotiable dimension as it is indicated by the patient's desire for a certain size. This is determined with the patient trying on sizers under a bra and a tight t-shirt serving as a "second skin" (Fig. 1.11). Once the patient determines the amount of projection that she wishes to have, the surgeon can then use that Z estimate to choose the corresponding X and Y for the implant based on her measurements and the type of implant she desires.

With the exception of very asymmetric cases, it is the authors' strong belief that the implants should be selected preoperatively during the consultation by the surgeon who is going to perform the surgery.

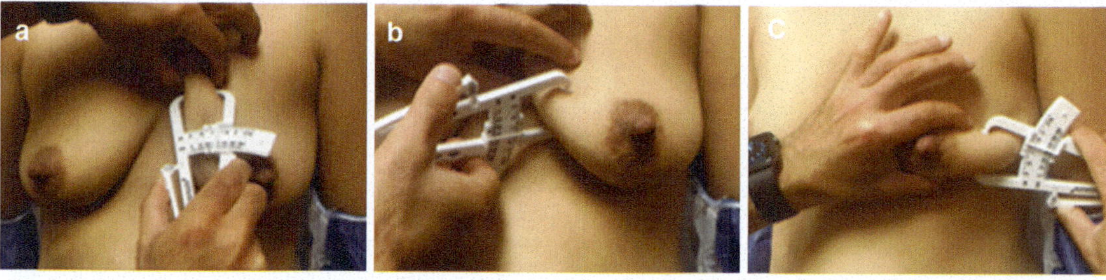

Fig. 1.8 Pinch tests of the breast measuring the upper pole (**a**), medial (**b**), and lateral thickness (**c**) of the breast

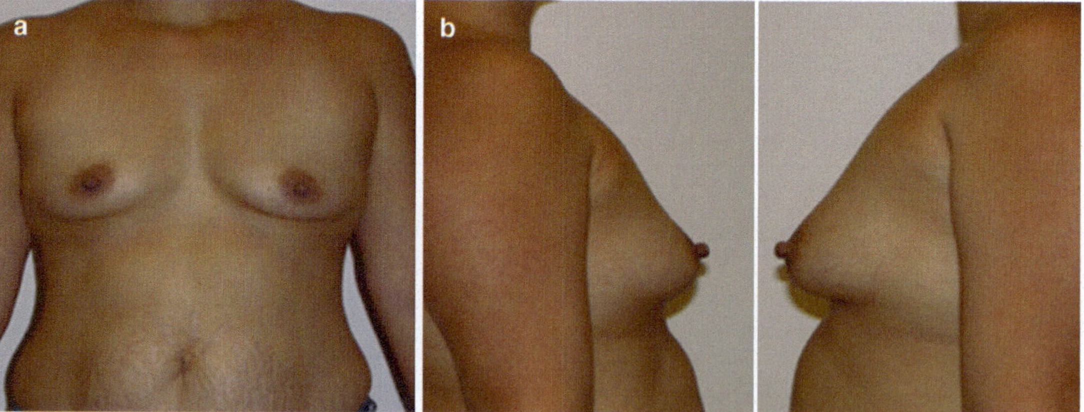

Fig. 1.9 This patient presents with a challenging anatomy. She has a wide X but a short Y, and a short lower pole (**a**). She is at high risk for double-bubble deformity and excessive upper pole fullness. Laterally, she has a different upper chest convexity that may influence the Z for each side (**b**)

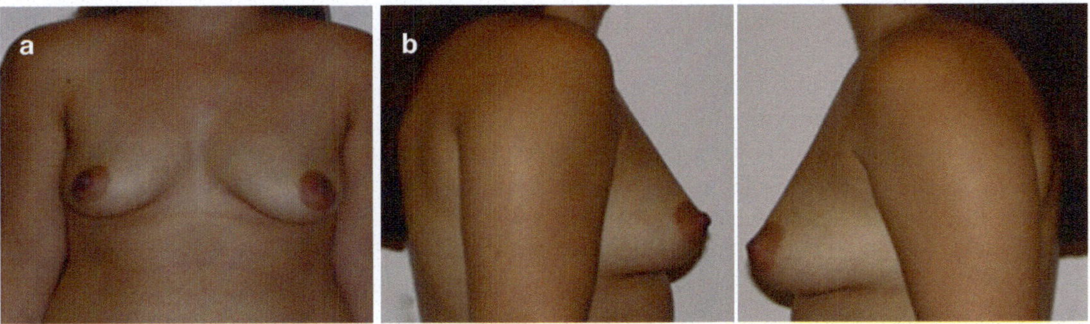

Fig. 1.10 This patient has a medium foot print that allows for more flexibility in implant selection in terms of *X*, *Y*, and *Z* (**a**, **b**)

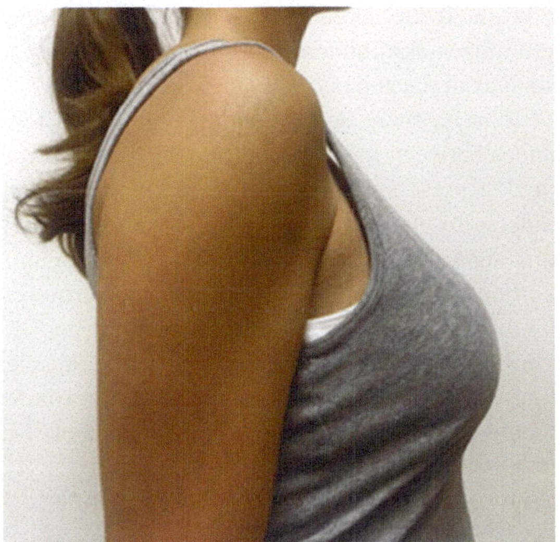

Fig. 1.11 Patient tries implant sizers preoperatively to determine the *Z* of the implant. The surgeon can then use that estimate to find the corresponding *X* and *Y* from the implant chart

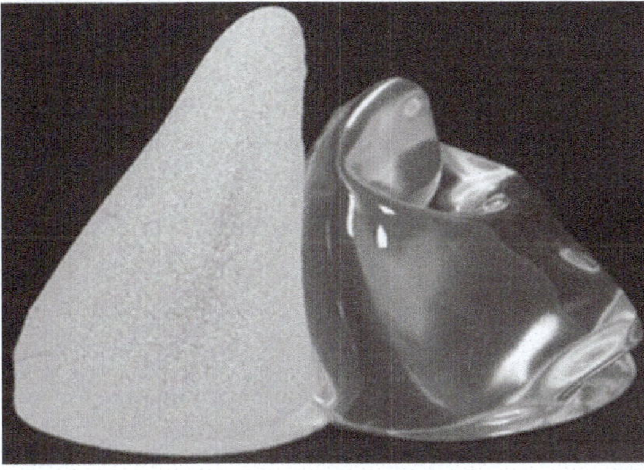

Fig. 1.12 A tear-shaped implant and soft gel (non–form stable) round implant side by side. Note that in the vertical position, the soft gel round implant takes on the "tear" shape

In general, tear-shaped implants have their advantages in cases where a certain shape is of more importance than just added volume, for example, for thin patients and breasts with a high footprint and shorter *Y* than *X*. On the other hand, the round implants with different cohesivities and fill ratios are preferred if a patient desires a more upper pole fullness with a round shape or does not want to have a textured implant. If a softer upper pole with a more tear-shaped appearance is desired but the patient does not want to use a textured implant, the authors recommend the use of a less cohesive and softer round gel implant that in the upright position takes on a more "tear shape" (Fig. 1.12).

One needs to remember that it is not about if a smooth, soft round implant can look like an anatomical implant with time; it is about if, when, and how with possible disadvantage of loss of pocket control. It is therefore the volume of distribution and not the cc of volume that dictates the implant selection and ultimately the shape of the breast.

It is an exciting time to be performing breast implant surgery because of the availability of a wide array of implants that can help solve many shape and asymmetry issues. The process of correct implant selection starts with a detailed physical exam, accurate biodimensional planning, and use of implant sizers during preoperative evaluation. In the authors' practice, all implants with their different characteristics are considered to tackle and solve minor to more difficult cases regarding breast and chest wall asymmetries in a way never presented before. Certain asymmetries are, however, not correctable, but it is vital to notice them and bring them to patient's attention preoperatively as it may have an influence on her final outcome.

Pocket Selection

The next step in the process is the pocket selection. The pinch test of the upper pole directs the surgeon in the choice of whether or not to place the implant subpectoral or prepectoral (subglandular/subfascial). Sufficient tissue coverage is important so that the implants do not become visible in the long run. Generally, at least 2 cm in the upper pole pinch test is desired for the prepectoral pocket. In the authors' practice, highly cohesive implants are thought to require more tissue coverage than less cohesive implants. This is perhaps due to the fact that more cohesive implant can stretch and shape the overlying tissue; however, due to its firmness it might also thin out the tissue overtime. In addition, the highly cohesive gel is more form stable and hence has a higher chance of visibility. Therefore, highly cohesive implants should more often be placed subpectoral.

Another potential difference in the pocket location is the rate of capsular contracture (CC). Although the exact cause (s) of CC is not well known, there is published data that suggest higher rate of CC in prepectoral versus subpectoral pocket. This, however, continues to be a source of debate, and more data are needed to settle the issue [29–33].

Opponents of prepectoral pocket selection also argue that the blood supply of the breast is altered for life, and this may have ramifications for the future breast surgeries. This point is less relevant if the surgeon recognizes this fact and minimizes skin undermining in repeat surgeries such as in mastopexy.

Finally, there are the biomechanical differences between the two pockets. The prepectoral pocket preserves the integrity of the pectoralis muscle by not requiring the division of its origin. As a result, there is no loss of strength and perhaps less pain in the long run. Furthermore, by avoiding the muscle, the prepectoral pocket eliminates the unfavorable forces of the muscle that cause animation deformity and contribute to the lateral and inferior displacement of the implants and double-bubble deformity [34] (Fig. 1.13).

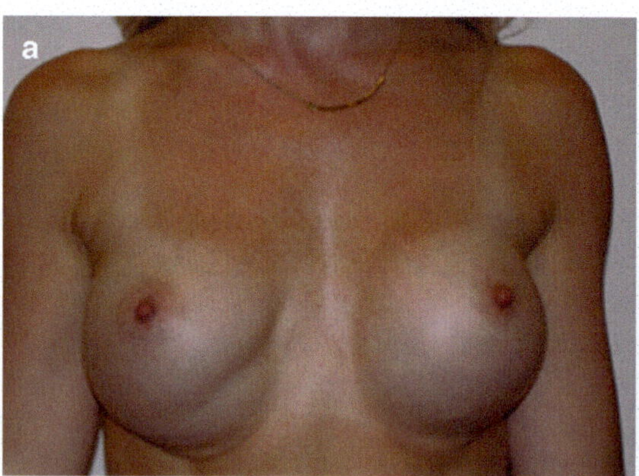

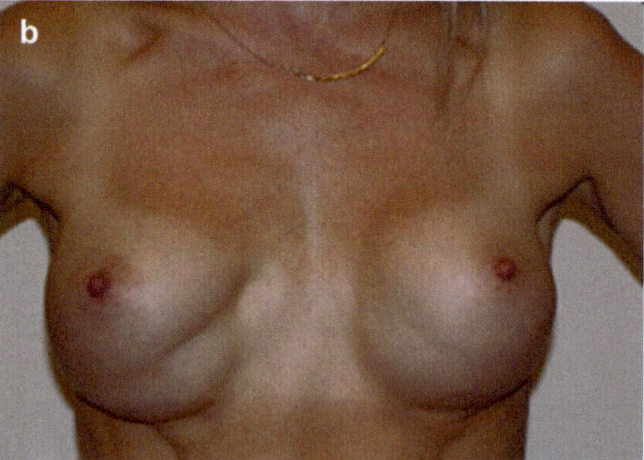

Fig. 1.13 Subpectoral augmentation with round gel implant complicated by double-bubble deformity and inferior malposition (**a**). Flexion of pectoralis major muscle can contribute to lateral malposition and double-bubble deformity (**b**)

Implant Surface Selection

The choice between smooth and textured surfaces is not a universally agreed upon topic, and there are many pros and cons for each device. The authors choose a wide variety of implants that are available dependent upon what the situation mandates. In general, the smooth round implants provide the following advantages: softer with more movement, decreased wrinkling with the new generation of highly cohesive and better fill ratio implants, less waterfall effect with glandular ptosis, and significantly less chance of BIA-ALCL. On the other hand, the smooth round implants have the following potential disadvantages: potential for higher capsular contracture, with rates as high as 3–5 times in the prepectoral pocket and 2 times in the subpectoral pocket in some studies, more lower pole stretching, less pocket stability and more malposition (uncontrolled tissue expansion), and less choices in varying the *X*, *Y*, and *Z* dimensions in certain cases [29–33]. The opposite holds true for the textured shaped implants.

One must remember that there is no holy grail of breast implants and different shaped implants, with different contents and surfaces can be great options in achieving good outcomes. It is more about patient selection and biodimensional planning.

Surgical Factors

Superficial Fascial System of the Breast

The understanding of the ligamentous and fascial system of the breast helps the surgeon to execute the surgical plan more accurately. The breast tissue (corpus mammae) is encased by two layers of fat and fascia, named the superficial fascia system of the breast (SFS) [35] (Fig. 1.14).

The SFS is divided into two layers: superficial and deep. The superficial layer covers the breast tissue anteriorly and deep layer covers it posteriorly. SFS layers coalesce with the deep fascia (covering the pectoralis muscle) in the periphery

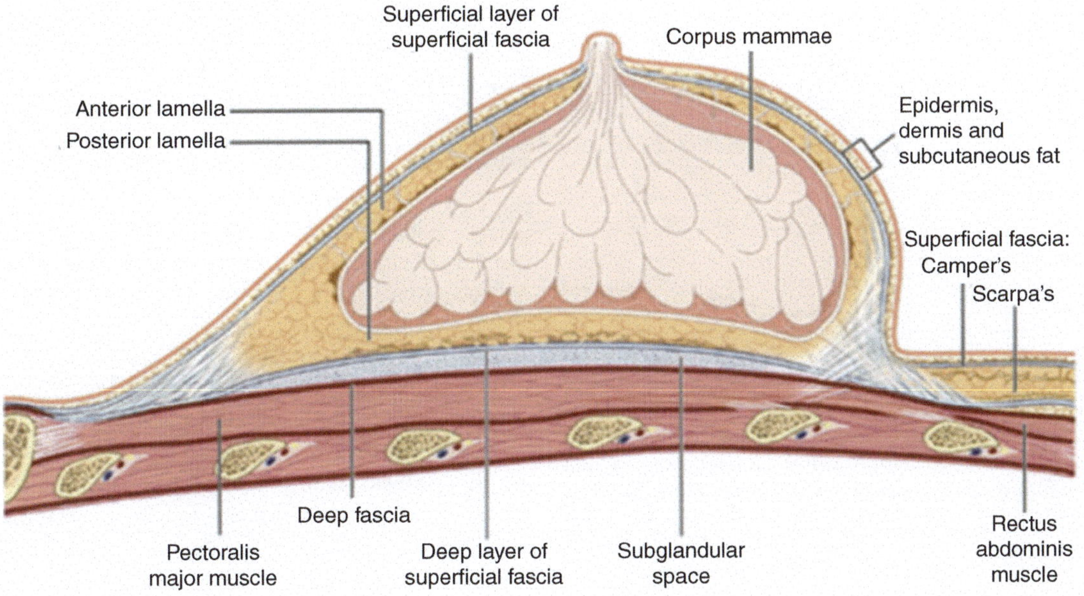

Fig. 1.14 Superficial fascial system; sagittal view. The corpus mammae is bounded by two layers of fascia and fat, the anterior and posterior lamina. (Copyright © Susan Gilbert. Used with permission)

of the breast forming a zone of adhesion called circummammary ligament. This zone is strongest along the IMF and sternal borders of the breast, and it is weakest along superior and lateral borders of breast (Fig. 1.15).

The circummammary ligament acts as the passage that arteries and nerves travel through on their way to the breast parenchyma and nipple areola complex. The Cooper's Ligaments are specialized vertical cutaneous ligaments that travel from the deep layer of SFS through the breast parenchyma and superficial layer of SFS to the dermis to anchor in the skin. This facilitates the connection between the breast tissue and the deep fascia via the circummammary ligament (Fig. 1.16).

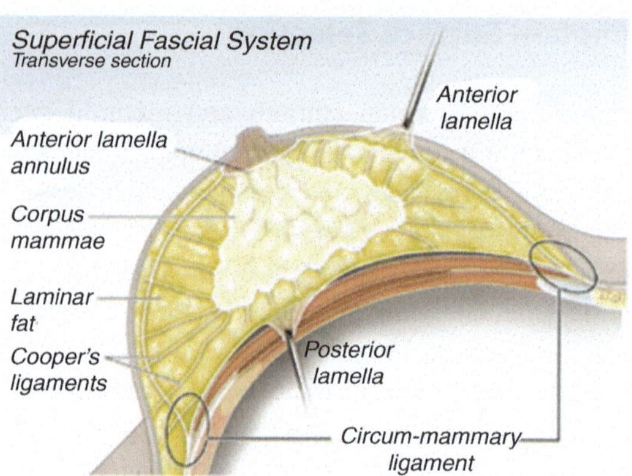

Fig. 1.16 Superficial fascial system; transverse section. The anterior and posterior lamina connect to the deep fascia of the chest wall in a circular zone of adhesion called the circummammary ligament, which connects the breast to the chest, providing support and structure to the breast. In addition, the Cooper's ligaments facilitate this connection and provide stability to the breast shape (Copyright © Susan Gilbert. Used with permission)

Preoperative Planning

As in any aesthetic surgical procedure, meticulous preoperative planning is essential. At the time of the preoperative visit, the surgeon must review patient's characteristics of her chest wall and existing breasts. Also, once again the surgical approach, pocket site, and selected implant are verified with the patient. The use of visual software is very beneficial in facilitating this process as it allows the patient to visually appreciate what the surgeon has in mind. In addition, the images can become part of the patient's documentation since many patients may not recall the conversations before the surgery (Fig. 1.17).

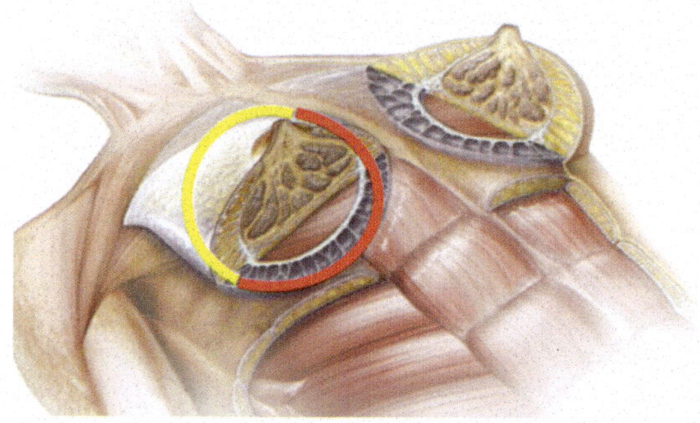

Fig. 1.15 Superficial fascial system; anterior and posterior lamina surround the corpus mammae, which can be seen erupting through an opening in the anterior lamina fat, the anterior lamina annulus. Note that the inframammary fold portion of the circummammary ligament (zone of adhesion) lies over the inscription between the rectus abdominis and pectoralis major muscle (circle). The zone of adhesion is strongest along the IMF and sternal borders of the breast (red hemicircle), and it is weakest along superior and lateral borders of breast (yellow hemicircle). (Modified from original. Copyright © Illumination Studios)

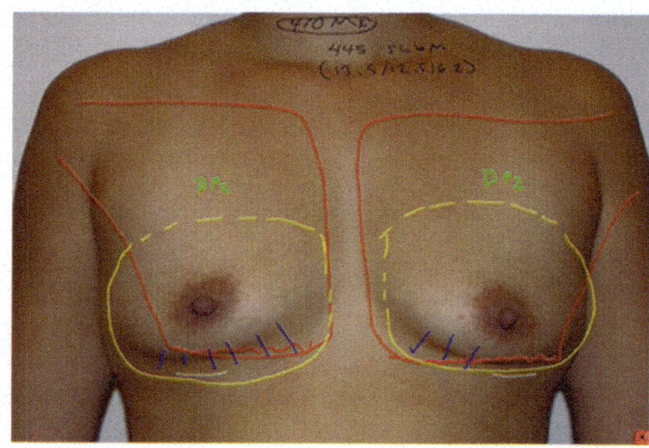

Fig. 1.17 Typical preoperative surgical planning that the authors create with the patient during the preoperative visit. These are documented as part of patient's chart. In addition, we use them in the operating room as a reminder for the surgical plan

Incision Site

There are four different incision locations for implant placement: inframammary fold, periareolar, transaxillary, and transumbilical approaches. For the authors, the preferred route of implant insertion is through an inframammary incision as this gives a very high level of control during pocket dissection and allows for simultaneous manual comparison of the pockets for symmetry. In addition, it minimizes the risk to areolar sensibility, interference with milk ducts, and thereby possible biofilm contamination of implants [36].

Marking

The beautification of the breast is in shaping the lower pole and not volumizing it. The most important step in achieving a beautiful result is the positioning of IMF, which in turn determines the nipple location. One must not think of nipple location to be at the center of the implant, rather the nipple position depends on the width of the implant and hence the width of breast:

$$\text{Breast width : Lower pole length} \simeq 2:1$$

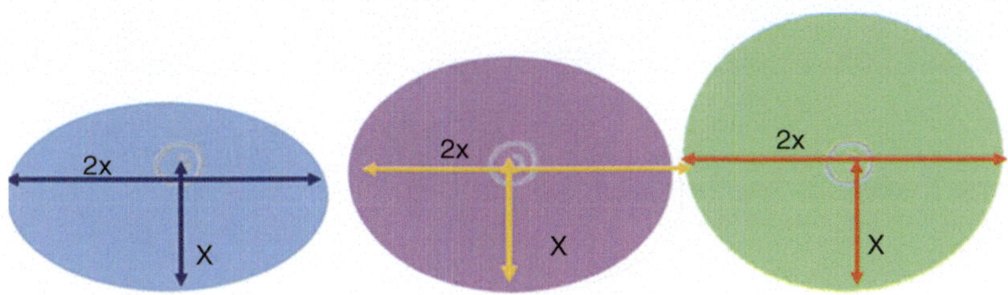

Placement of the inframammary skin incision is the most important step in achieving this goal because that is where the final IMF will be. This may require a possible lowering of the inframammary fold which depends on the N-IMF distance, the width of the implant, and the patient's tissue characteristics (Fig. 1.18).

In general, the wider the implant, the lower the fold needs to be. We follow an algorithmic approach to the placement of the IMF incision: the base width of the implant generates a corresponding value for the new N-IMF distance under maximum tension, which then becomes the site of the new position of the inframammary fold and thereby the inframammary incision (Fig. 1.19).

The algorithmic approach is, however, different for the textured versus smooth implants and is generated based on experiences with textured and smooth implants [37] (Tables 1.1 and 1.2).

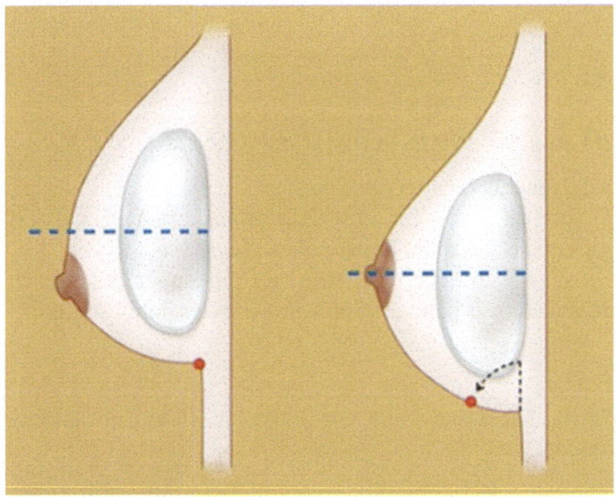

Fig. 1.18 (Left) Implant placement in a patient with a short crease-to-areola distance is suboptimal if the crease is not released. The nipple position will appear low and the upper pole excessively full. (Right) Release and lowering of the crease to center the implant on the nipple position produces optimal aesthetics. (Used with permission of Wolters Kluwer Health, Inc., from Rehnke et al. [35])

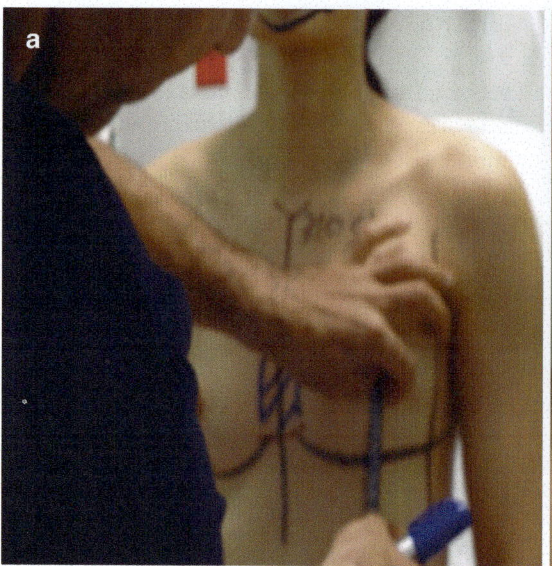

Fig. 1.19 Surgical marking for IMF incision. The new IMF and hence the incision site is determined by measuring the N:IMF distance under maximum tension (**a**) and placing the incision at the desired site based on the algorithm in Tables 1.1 and 1.2 (**b**)

Table 1.1 Guidelines for lowering IMF for textured implants (Randquist)

Base diameter	Distance to new IMF (nipple on stretch)
11.5 cm	8.0 cm
12.0 cm	8.5 cm
12.5 cm	9.0 cm
13.0 cm	9.5 cm
13.5 cm	10 cm (never more)

Adjustments for individual patients:

Subtract 0.5 cm for loose skin, prepectoral position or if patient desires more upper pole fullness

Add 0.5 cm for tight skin, >3 cm upper pole pinch thickness or if patient desires more lower pole fullness

Table 1.2 Guidelines for lowering IMF for smooth implants

Base diameter	Distance to new IMF (nipple on stretch)
11.5 cm	7 cm
12.0 cm	7.5 cm
12.5 cm	8 cm
13.0 cm	8.5 cm
13.5 cm	9 cm (never more)

Adjustments for individual patients:

Subtract 0.5 cm for loose skin, prepectoral position or if patient desires more upper pole fullness

Add 0.5 cm for tight skin, >3 cm upper pole pinch thickness or if patient desires more lower pole fullness

The lowering of the fold is more for a textured implant than a smooth implant with the same content and volume due to different amount of tissue expansion. As mentioned above, the highly cohesive textured form stable gel implants in a precise pocket, work as controlled tissue expanders. As such, depending on how the volume of gel is distributed in the implant, it will apply tissue expansion and skin stretch where most of the gel is distributed. Once the cohesive gel implant has expanded the tissue in accordance to predesigned shape, it does not influence or alter the breast shape or positioning anymore over time. In contrast, the smooth implants have less control over the skin and tissue expansion and continue to do so by following the gravity, going downward in standing and toward the axilla in supine. Therefore, lowering the IMF for the smooth implant is done more conservatively.

For example, an implant with 12 cm would require a nipple to fold distance of 7.5 cm or 8.5 cm (±0.5 cm) for smooth or textured implants, respectively. For each 0.5 cm increase in implant base width, 0.5 cm is added to the amount necessary for potential lowering and for each 0.5 cm decrease in implant base width, 0.5 cm is subtracted from the amount of IMF lowering. In addition, if the patient has approximately >3 cm of parenchyma in the lower pole, an additional 0.5 cm should be added to the distance the IMF is to be lowered. Furthermore, if the patient has a tight, firm skin envelope that does not stretch, as often is the case in patients with aplasia mammae or constricted lower pole, 0.5 cm should be added to the lowering amount. In patients with a loose overstretched skin as seen in patients with postpartum or post massive weight loss breasts, 0.5 cm should be subtracted. The system can also be adjusted according to the surgeon's or the patient's aesthetic preference regarding more or less upper and lower pole fullness.

Note that implants with the same *X* but different *Z* require the IMF incision at the same level. This is due to the fact that more projection simply means more gel distributed anteriorly and not inferiorly. The increased gel anteriorly applies more expanding energy and thereby stretches the curved anterior surface of the breast. This elongates the curvilinear N:IMF distance proportionally along the surface of the lower half while keeping the linear N:IMF distance the same.

With the level of skin incision decided and marked, the height and width of the implant should be outlined on the patient's chest wall (Fig. 1.20).

It is important to respect the medial attachments of the major pectoral muscle in order to prevent possible implant visibility or symmastia. Of note, if a patient desire more cleavage and has the appropriate >2 cm upper pole pinch, the surgeon may consider the prepectoral plane as this medial dissection is not limited by the pectoral muscle. Yet, one must consider that there is still a medial limitation by the circummammary ligament. Laterally, the pocket must be developed to accommodate the *X* dimension of the implant. This is a very important point in creating pocket stability. As described earlier, the circummammary ligament is the weakest superiorly and laterally and over dissection beyond the diameter of the implant will result in loss of pocket control and lateral malposition.

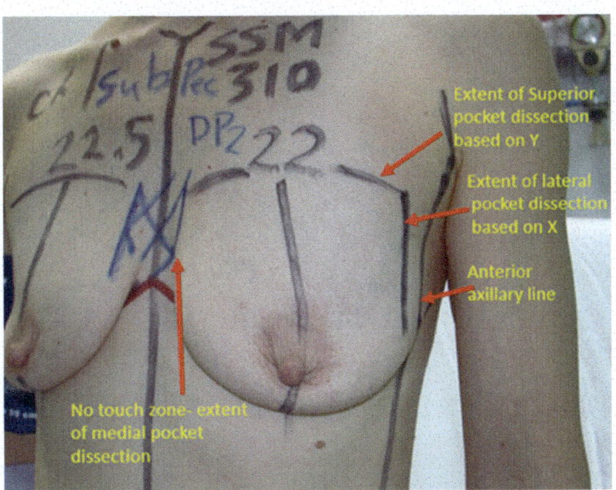

Fig. 1.20 Surgical marking for breast augmentation. The *X* and *Y* of the implant are marked on the skin. Note that the *X* is measured from "no touch" zone medially and toward the anterior axillary line laterally. In a moderate size breast, the *X* is narrower than the actual breast width that extends to the anterior axillary line. The pocket dissection must stay limited to the external marking in order to minimize violation of SFS and avoid malposition

Adhering to these basic principles should result in a perfect placement of the implants. After the preoperative planning and a thorough measuring and marking of the patient's chest wall, the patient is ready for surgery.

Surgery

The patient is placed in the supine position with arms padded and secured on the arm boards in semi-abducted fashion at 80°. We use outpatient general anesthesia with laryngeal mask airway although it can also be done under sedation.

With the patient anesthetized, a rectangular area reaching cranially just above the clavicles, laterally to the dorsal axillary line and caudally to the umbilicus, is scrubbed using 10% chlorhexidine solution. After patient is draped and draped, nipple shields are applied.

Before proceeding with the surgery, the surgeon now double-checks the N-IMF distance under maximum stretch (Fig. 1.21). Checking the N-IMF distance is at times more easily done on the operating table as it requires an upward pull of the nipple, which in some patients is painful.

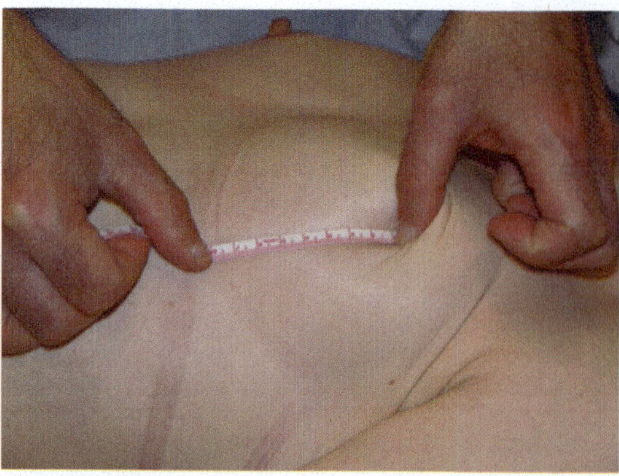

Fig. 1.21 Remeasuring N:IMF distance under maximum tension on the operating table to verify the location of IMF incision and the new IMF

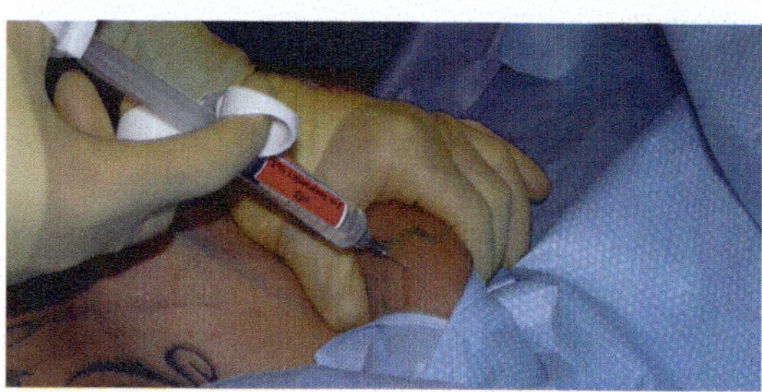

Fig. 1.22 As part of breast injection with local anesthesia, the axillary tail of the pectoralis is injected. This is done by pinching the muscle origin near the shoulder with the nondominant fingers and while injecting into the muscle

To reduce postoperative pain approximately 20 cc of 0.25% Marcaine and 1% lidocaine with 1:100,000 epinephrine is injected per breast deep into the upper portion of each major pectoral muscle and around the breast and incision site (Fig. 1.22).

The following section first describes the authors' breast augmentation procedure for the subpectoral pocket dissection and implant insertion through an inframammary incision. After this follows a description of the prepectoral implant placement. For the best visualization and ergonomics for the surgeon, all surgeries should be performed from each side of the operating table for the corresponding breast with the surgeon in a sitting position wearing a headlight while keeping his/her spine and the neck supported and in neutral position. For the optimal view of the pocket, the patient's bed is airplaned side to side and the height of the bed adjusted.

The surgical procedure of breast augmentation can be divided into eight different steps as follows:

1. Skin incision, dissection through the deep dermis, subcutaneous fat, and superficial fascia system
2. Identification of the major pectoral muscle – entrance into the subpectoral space
3. Creation of the subpectoral implant pocket
4. Implant insertion
5. Wound closure
6. Dressing

Skin Incision

An incision is made according to the preoperative markings using a sharp scalpel. As discussed above, the preferred placement of the scar is in the planned inframammary fold, which may or may not be the same as the existing fold. The length of the incision depends on the size of the implant. A 3.5 cm long incision is sufficient for a 300-cc implant, and a 4-cm-long incision is sufficient for a 400-cc implant. If necessary, the incision should be made wider in order for the implant to be inserted easily without the risk of shell or gel rupture.

The incision is made through the epidermis and into the superficial dermis sharply. At this point, the surgeon changes to the guarded electrocautery in order to avoid unnecessary bleeding.

Identification of the Major Pectoral Muscle

Using the guarded electrocautery, the dissection continues down through the dermis and then in a cephalad direction through the subcutaneous fat and superficial fascia system until the pectoralis major muscle is identified (Fig. 1.23).

As soon as the muscle becomes visible, dissection is continued along the inferolateral border

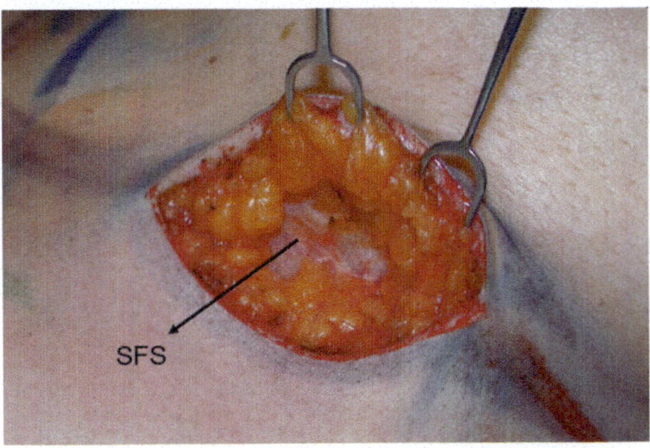

Fig. 1.23 The IMF incision through the skin and subcutaneous layer. Note the well-defined SFS layer

of the muscle while retracting the tissue anteriorly. The objective is to identify the areolar space between the pectoralis major and minor muscles since the only structure that gets lifted is the pectoralis major muscle. The upward retraction of the breast tissue is the key as this will concomitantly elevates the pectoralis major muscle away from the other muscles. This maneuver is facilitated due to the presence of suspensory Cooper's ligaments that connect the deep fascia of the pectoralis major muscle and the breast parenchyma via the SFS layers (see Fig. 1.16). It is imperative to not cut the muscle inferiorly unless you can elevate the muscle off the chest wall and away from the nearby muscles. Inability to elevate the pectoralis muscle most likely indicates that the identified muscle is actually not the pectoralis major, but rather the serratus, rectus, intercostal muscle, or pectoralis minor muscles. Once the lateral border of the pectoralis major is identified, the fascia is incised to expose the underlying muscle. Although this is usually not a difficult task, one must be aware of some variation to the anatomy of the origin of the pectoralis major muscle from the ribs and its interdigitation with the underlying pectoralis minor muscle. Unless the areolar space between the two muscles is clearly identified, the submuscular dissection should be held off until further clarification. One maneuver that helps with this situation is to continue cephalad along the lateral border of the pectoralis muscle with electrocautery while retracting the tissue anteriorly under tension until the space between the two muscles becomes clear.

Creation of the Implant Pocket

The main objective during the pocket dissection is to create a pocket that is optimal in size with regard to *X* and *Y* of the selected implant. The width of the pocket is determined by a correct dissection in both the lateral and medial directions. Similarly, the height of the pocket is determined by precise dissection in both the inferior and superior directions.

At this point, we use the monopolar cautery forceps (Marina Medical) to enter the submuscular space and begin the division of the origin of the pectoralis fibers 5 mm anterior to the chest wall (Fig. 1.24). With the needlepoint forceps in the closed position, using a blended cut and coagulation current, continue dissection medially to the sternum and inferiorly to the desired inframammary fold level. The advantages of using the monopolar cautery are a bloodless dissection and less muscle contraction, therefore affording the surgeon the accuracy and the precision needed to perform the dissection more efficiently and safely.

Leaving a thin strip of muscle fibers at the insertion prevents blood vessels within the muscle, often intercostal perforators, from retracting into the underlying tissue.

The pocket dissection follows a standard circular pattern under direct visualization with either headlight illumination or lighted retractor (Fig. 1.25).

It continues medially and then cranially along the medial and superior borders of the pocket before it is completed laterally in a caudal direction toward the inferolateral border of the pocket. At all times, the retractor should be moved forward and repositioned further and further under the pectoralis major muscle while retracting the muscle anteriorly. The retractor is constantly

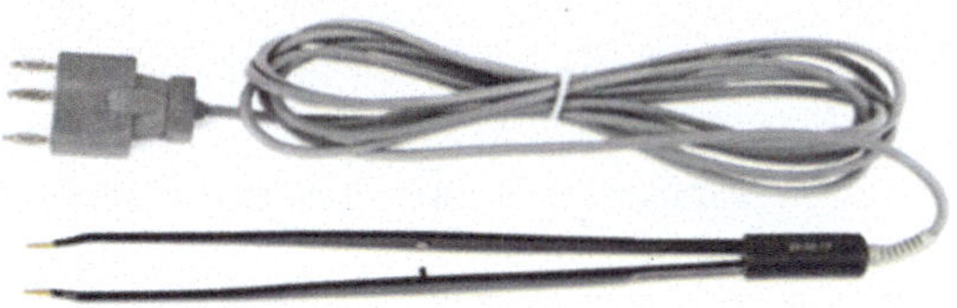

Fig. 1.24 Marina Medical Monopolar forceps

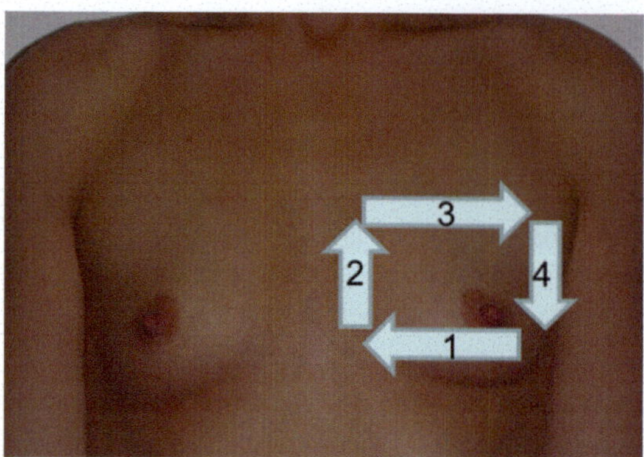

Fig. 1.25 The standard circular pattern of pocket dissection

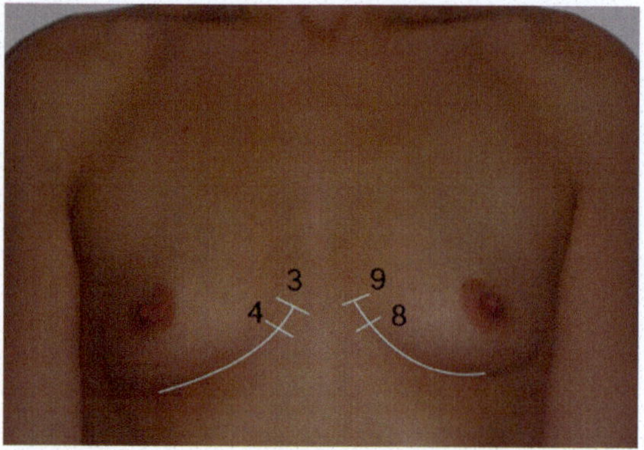

Fig. 1.26 The extent of full thickness pectoralis muscle release is to the 4 o'clock on the right and 8 o'clock on the left side. The muscle is further thinned out to 3 o'clock on the right and 9 o'clock on the left side

kept firmly elevated in order to help continuous identification of the pectoralis major muscle and avoiding any contact with the perichondrium. Furthermore, the blade of the retractor should be inserted completely into the pocket under the muscle and the muscle should not be folded on top of the blade.

The medial dissection is preferably performed using a sweeping motion with the electrocautery forceps in a craniocaudal direction. This facilitates early visualization of blood vessels, including perforators, which then can be cauterized before they are cut. Complete release of the pectoralis major muscle's abdominal and caudal sternocostal insertions are performed to about 4 o'clock on the patient's right side and to about 8 o'clock on the patient's left side. Dissection and release of these lower muscle insertions is essential in order for the implant to be positioned properly in a caudo-medial direction. The inside surface of the pocket should be made completely even, as any unevenness could cause visible indentions in the tissue. It must be emphasized that the bulk of the medial attachments of the muscle, cranial to the above described 4 and 8 o'clock levels should not under any circumstances be completely divided except for the transition zones where the muscle is thinned out to the 3 o'clock on the right side and 9 o'clock on the left side to create a smooth transition especially if she has thick muscle (Figs. 1.26 and 1.27).

There are usually accessary muscle fibers that must also be divided in order to create a smooth transition all along the medial border of the pocket without any step offs. Over dissection and release of fibers medially will not correct a very wide intermammary space; it only increases

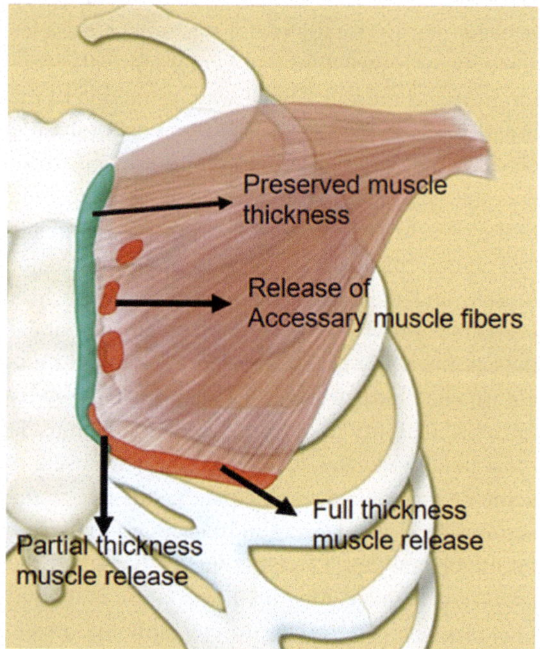

Fig. 1.27 Submuscular pocket creation. Note the zones of complete muscle release (red) and preserved muscle fibers (green) with the transition zone in between where only partial muscle release has been done. The release of accessary fibers is required to create a uniform pocket. (Modified with permission of Wolters Kluwer Health, Inc., from Rehnke et al. [35])

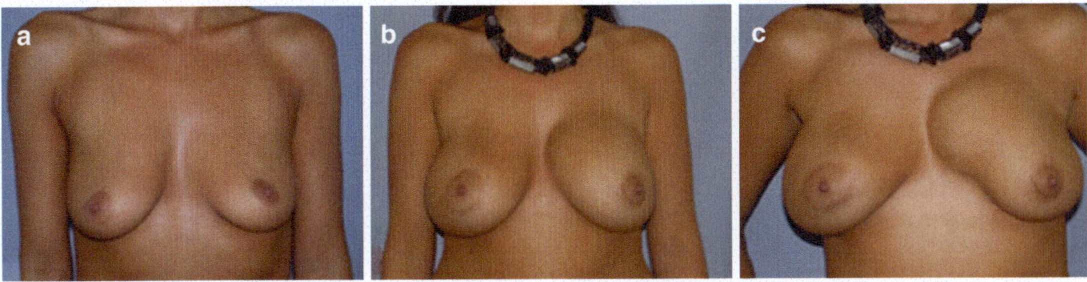

Fig. 1.28 This patient underwent dual plane I dissection with overzealous medial muscle fiber release on the left side. Preoperative picture (**a**). Postoperative picture demonstrating the disinsertion of the medial fibers medially at rest (**b**) and with muscle flexion (**c**)

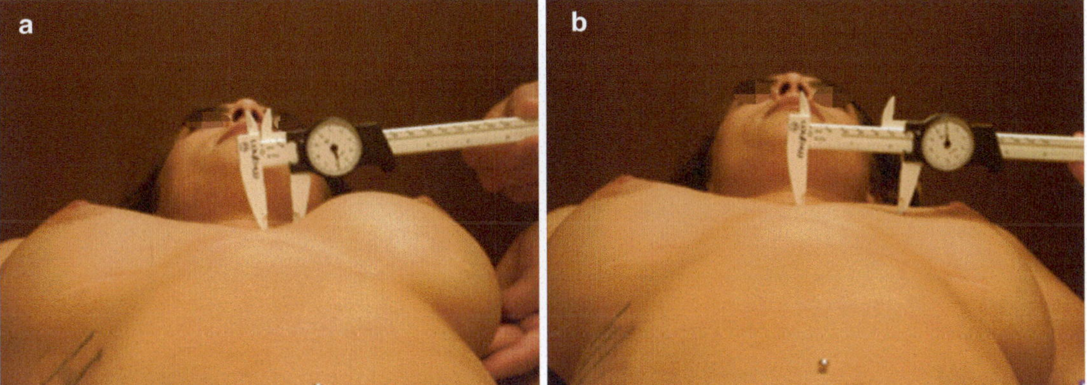

Fig. 1.29 Lateral malposition of the breast implants. No lateral movement of left implant with lateral manual support (**a**) and a 5 cm lateral malposition of the left implant without manual support in supine position (**b**)

the risk of future implant visibility, mediocranial implant displacement, and symmastia (Fig. 1.28).

Similarly, over dissection superiorly can result in cranial displacement of the implants as the tissue in the upper part of the pocket including the circummammary ligament is very loose.

Lateral over dissection should also be avoided by respecting the external preoperative surgical marking. The surgeon should not dissect beyond the necessary width needed to accommodate the *X* of the implant. Once again, it should be noted that the anterior axillary line and lateral extent of the pocket may not be concordant. To verify the extent of lateral dissection, the surgeon can use a ruler by placing it abutted to the medial most aspect of the pocket and measuring laterally to the desired width (*X* of the selected implant). This maneuver is especially helpful in revision or reconstructive cases where creating lateral control is of utmost importance. Also, be reminded that the SFS is the weakest laterally. Ignoring this key point will create too wide of a pocket with heightened risk of malposition laterally (Fig. 1.29).

This completes dual plane I dissection. After the dissection has been performed on both sides, the surgeon should take time to palpate both pockets simultaneously using the index fingers, ensuring that all surfaces are even, that the pockets are wide enough, and that the tissue release in the anterior direction is sufficient (Fig. 1.30).

At this point, if there are any tight bands of tissue palpated anteriorly in the lower pole, radial release is performed using the electrocautery. Radial release is also indicated in cases of lowering IMF, constricted bases, and tuberous breast. As mentioned earlier, IMF is the fusion of the deep fascia attached to the pectoralis mus-

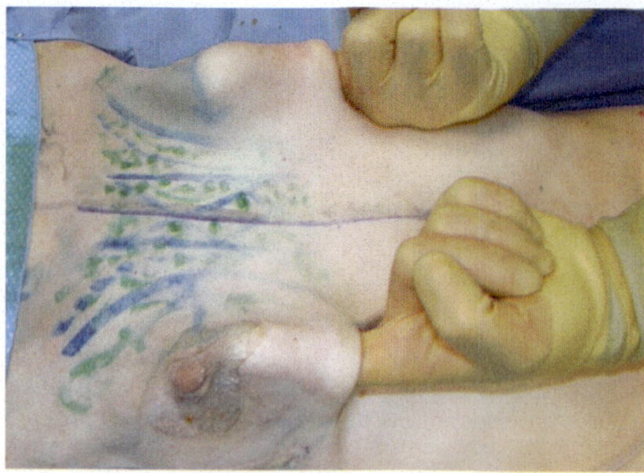

Fig. 1.30 At the completion of the pocket creation, simultaneous bimanual palpation is important to verify symmetrical pocket creation and check for any tight bands

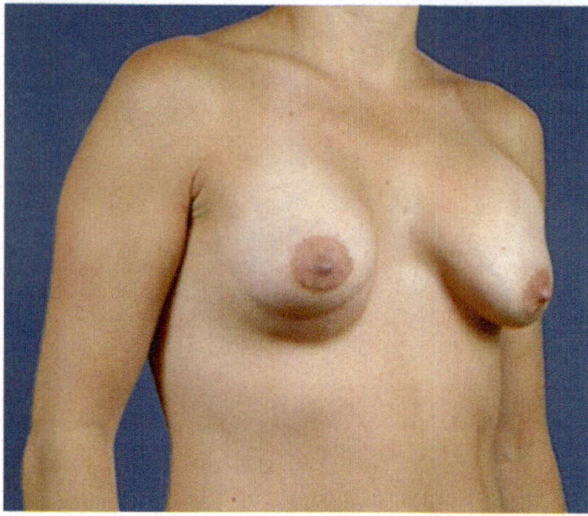

Fig. 1.31 Double-bubble deformity due to preservation of the native fold

cle and the SFS of the breast. If IMF lowering in the subpectoral pocket is required, one must transition into a more superficial subglandular plane above the pectoralis fascia. Dissection deep to the pectoral fascia will likely result in a lowered fold with persistence of the native fold structure, resulting in a double-bubble deformity (Figs. 1.31 and 1.32).

Finally, if the preoperative plan included dual plane II or III dissection, it is performed at this time. The indications for dual plane II or III are constricted bases, tuberous breast, and glandular ptosis. The purpose of increased dual plane dissection is to bring more of the breast tissue in the lower pole in contact with the implant and facilitate the desired lower pole shaping. To perform dual plane II, the surgeon releases the freed origin of the muscle inferiorly from the breast parenchyma in a subfascial plane (to minimize bacterial contamination and preserve the Cooper's ligaments attachment on pectoralis fascia) using electrocautery for about 1 cm or to a point corresponding to the lower edge of the areola. Dual plane III is created if this release is continued to a level corresponding to above the areola (Figs. 1.33 and 1.34).

Implant Insertion

Before the implants are inserted, it is imperative to make sure that absolutely no bleeding is present in either of the implant pockets. The pockets are irrigated with triple antibiotics, which is a mixture of 1 g of cefazolin sodium, 80 mg gentamycin, 50 cc betadine mixed in 500 mL of normal saline. At this point, the incision is prepped with betadine gel, the surgeon changes to a new pair of gloves and is careful not to touch anything except the implants during insertion. The implant box is opened and while the implants are still in the sterile box, each box is injected with 60 cc of antibiotic irrigation (Fig. 1.35).

To introduce the implant into the pocket, it is best to use a sleeve or Keller funnel (Allergan, Inc., Irvine, CA) to minimize contact with the skin (no touch technique) (Fig. 1.36).

For the tear-shaped implants, the implant should be inserted with the apex first. The incision should be sufficiently wide in order for

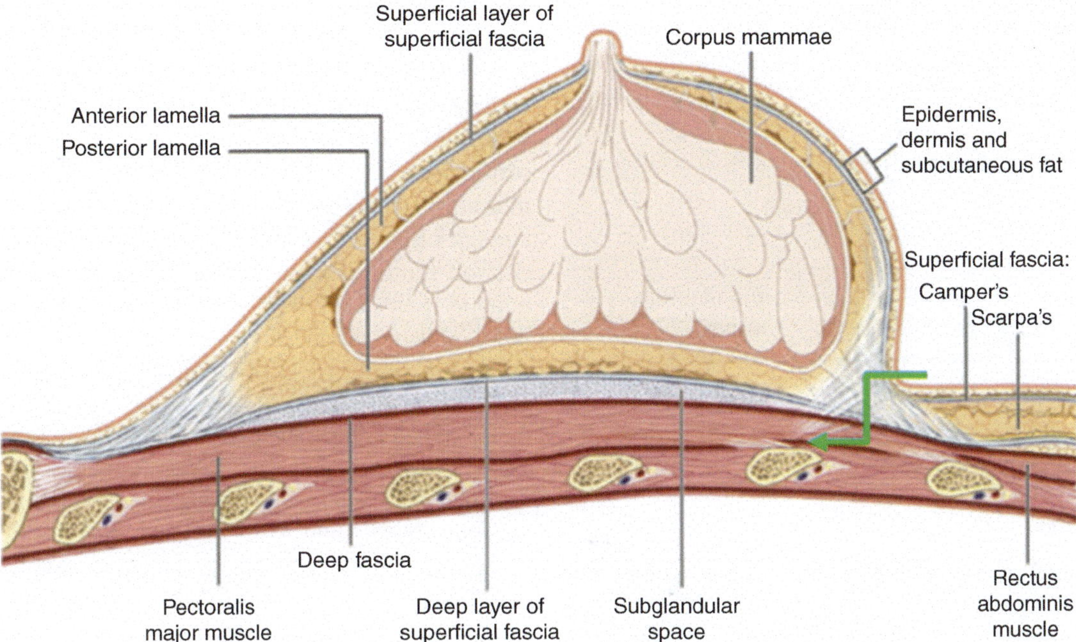

Fig. 1.32 If subpectoral pocket with lowering of the IMF is intended, the native IMF must be disrupted to minimize the risk of double-bubble deformity. The course of dissection from the new site of IMF to the subpectoral pocket is depicted in green arrow. (Modified and used with permission. Copyright © Susan Gilbert)

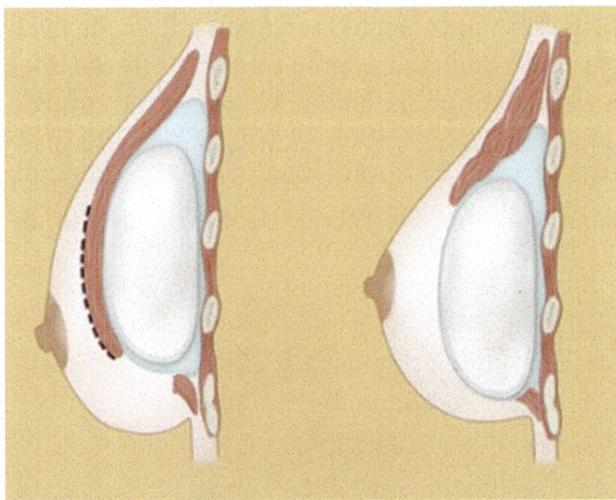

Fig. 1.33 The release of pectoralis origin in dual plane I–III dissection juxtaposes the implant to the breast parenchyma, which stimulates lower pole expansion. (Used with permission of Wolters Kluwer Health, Inc., from Rehnke et al. [35])

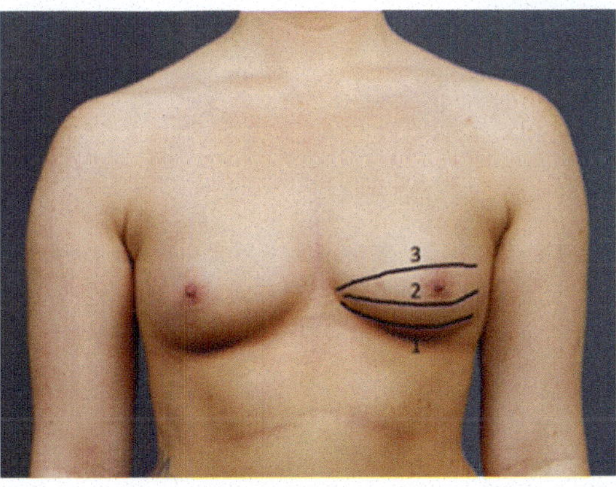

Fig. 1.34 Dual plane I–III and its corresponding level on the breast

the implant to be inserted easily, as mentioned above. If the implant is inserted using excessive force, this might cause fracturing of the gel.

Once the implant has been inserted, its correct position should be verified. This is done by palpating or visualizing the markings on the ventral, caudal surface of the tear-shaped implants, or posterior surface of the round implants. The implant's position in the pocket medially, lat-

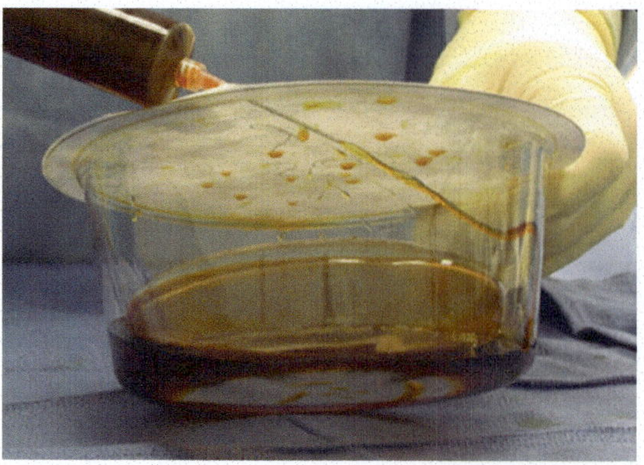

Fig. 1.35 Injection of 60 cc of antibiotic mixture into the sterile implant box while the box is still sealed. The implant will remain in the sealed box until the time of insertion

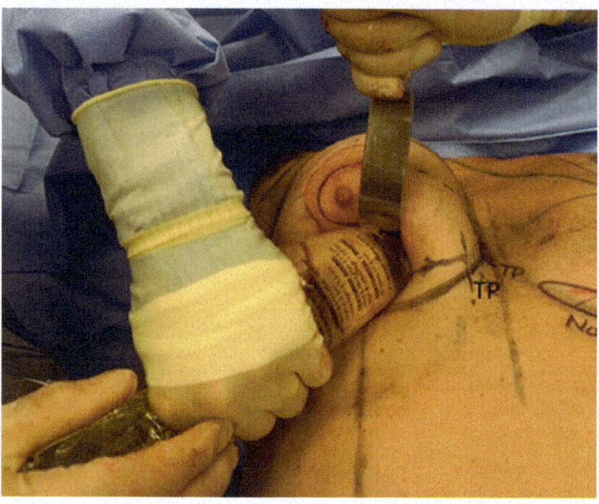

Fig. 1.36 Insertion of implant into the pocket using "no touch" technique and a sleeve

erally, and cranially is also checked. If the pocket seems too tight on either side, or if there are strands of tissue causing indentions in the implant, this is corrected. The surgeon should always strive toward performing perfect primary pocket dissection, which does not require any corrections once the implant has been inserted. No sizers (with rare exceptions in cases of severe asymmetry or for the novice surgeon) or drains are necessary, as these cause untoward traumatization and increase the risk of bacterial contamination.

Wound Closure

A correctly performed wound closure is crucial, and this step of the procedure should also be performed in a standardized fashion. Wound closure serves several functions. As described below, a multilayer closing technique that adapts a large amount of tissue over the wound minimizes the risk of future implant visibility. Furthermore, juxtaposition of the tissue of lower pole against the implant enhances the controlled tissue expansion where most of action–reaction takes place. In addition, anchoring the wound to the thoracic wall defines the new inframammary fold and places the scar directly in the inframammary fold. This is especially important in cases of lowered IMF.

The wound is closed in three layers as follows. First a deep layer with three 2-0 absorbable sutures is made. To place these sutures accurately, the surgeon determines and marks the location of the desired IMF fixation by palpating the base of the bilateral IMF inside the wound (Fig. 1.37).

The needle is passed through the tissue of the chest wall surface at the level of the desired IMF. It is important to get a good grip in the muscle fascia and musculature so that the thread does not cut through the tissue. However, the surgeon must be careful not to go too deep avoiding the risk of injuries to the intercostal neurovascular bundles along the inferior border of rib and the

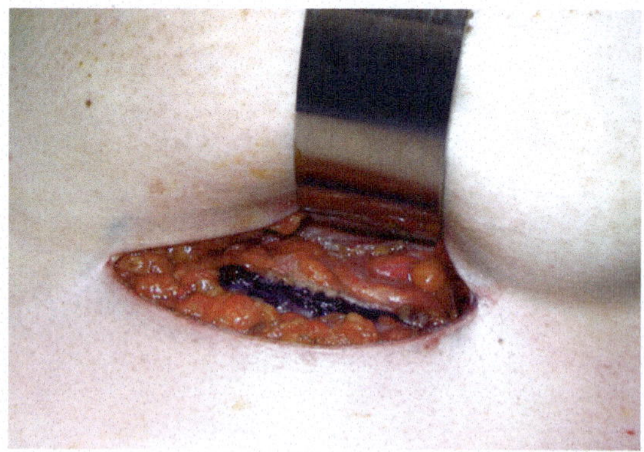

Fig. 1.37 The site of the desired IMF fixation sutures is palpated on both sides and marked

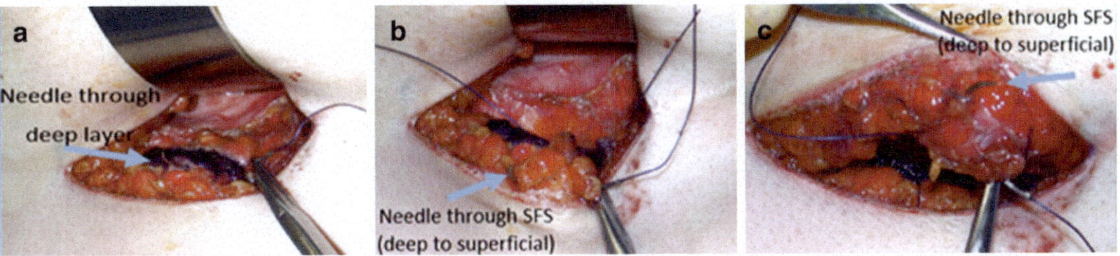

Fig. 1.38 IMF fixation suture. Suture purchase of deep layer (**a**) and inferior (**b**)/superior (**c**) SFS from deep to superficial directions on both sides

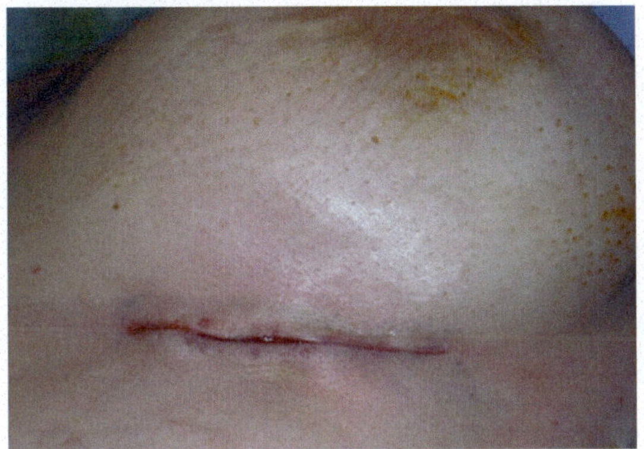

Fig. 1.39 Everted edges of the skin after placement of IMF fixation sutures

pleura. The amount of available tissue depends on the constitution of the patient, and a superficial grip in the periosteum might be needed in a very thin patient. This may cause additional postoperative pain with breathing, but it is a better alternative for the long-term durability. The needle is subsequently passed through the deep layers of fat and SFS on both sides of the wound from deep to superficial direction before the knot is tied (Fig. 1.38).

When placed correctly, this first row of sutures will approximate the edges of the wound (Fig. 1.39).

The next layer of sutures serves to approximate the wound edges further and to bring tissue into an everted crest on both sides of the wound. A two-layer closure of deep dermis and subcuticular layers is done using barbed double-ended 2-0 Monoderm Quill sutures.

Dressing

The incision is then sealed with surgical glue. A single layer of tape is then applied to the incision as the only dressing, which will be removed by the patient after 1 week. No drain is necessary for the primary cases.

Prepectoral Implant Placement

If the patient has sufficient tissue coverage (upper pole pinch test of ≥2 cm) and wants to avoid pectoralis involvement, or has a major desire of cleavage, the implants can be placed prepectorally. The dissection of the prepectoral pocket is performed on top of the major pectoral muscle in either subglandular or subfascial (deep to the pectoralis fascia) plane (Fig. 1.40). The subfascial plane theoretically provides a layer of protection between the implant and breast parenchyma and hence reduces the exposure to biofilm contamination [38, 39]. In theory, this may help reduce the risk of capsular contracture. In our opinion, the subfascial pocket provides more advantages (preserved integrity of pectoralis muscle and its strength, preservation of Cooper's ligaments, potentially lower risk of biofilm contamination, no animation deformity, no unfavorable forces exerted by the pectoralis muscle on the implant, easier recovery, and less long-term pain issues) than disadvantages (more visibility of implant and rippling and possibly more potential for capsular contracture) and therefore has become our preferred method of augmentation in the right patient. The dissection in the prepectoral pocket must once again follow the same principle of pocket development in accordance with the dimensions of the implant that has been chosen in order to keep the pocket tight and minimize the risk of implant malposition. In addition, if the IMF lowering is planned, the inferior portion of circummammary ligament (IMF) must be divided with radial release in order to avoid double-bubble deformity. For the subfascial pocket, this is accomplished by transitioning the dissection into the subglandular pocket near the IMF incision as the attachments creating the fold are superficial to the deep pectoral fascia (Fig. 1.41). The lowering of IMF in the subglandular pocket is more easily achieved as the subglandular plane dissection inferiorly is in the appropriate plane to lower and obliterate the native fold (Fig. 1.42).

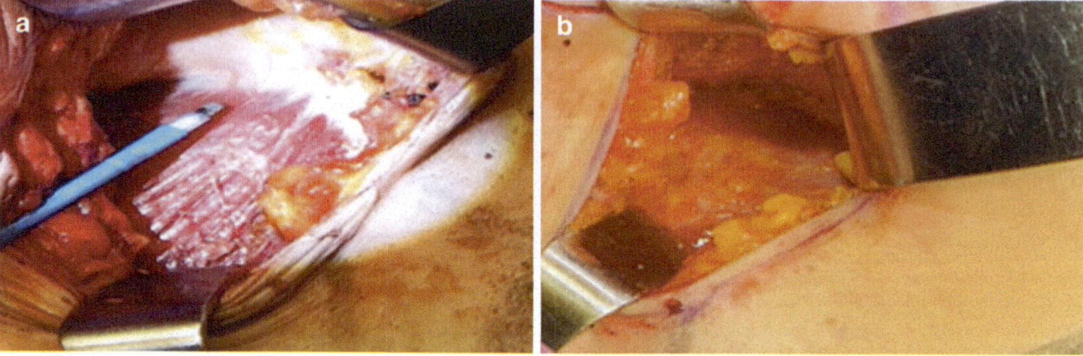

Fig. 1.40 Subfascial (**a**) and subglandular (**b**) prepectoral pocket development. The fascia albeit thin is in fact well defined and can potentially help keep the surgeon out of the breast parenchyma

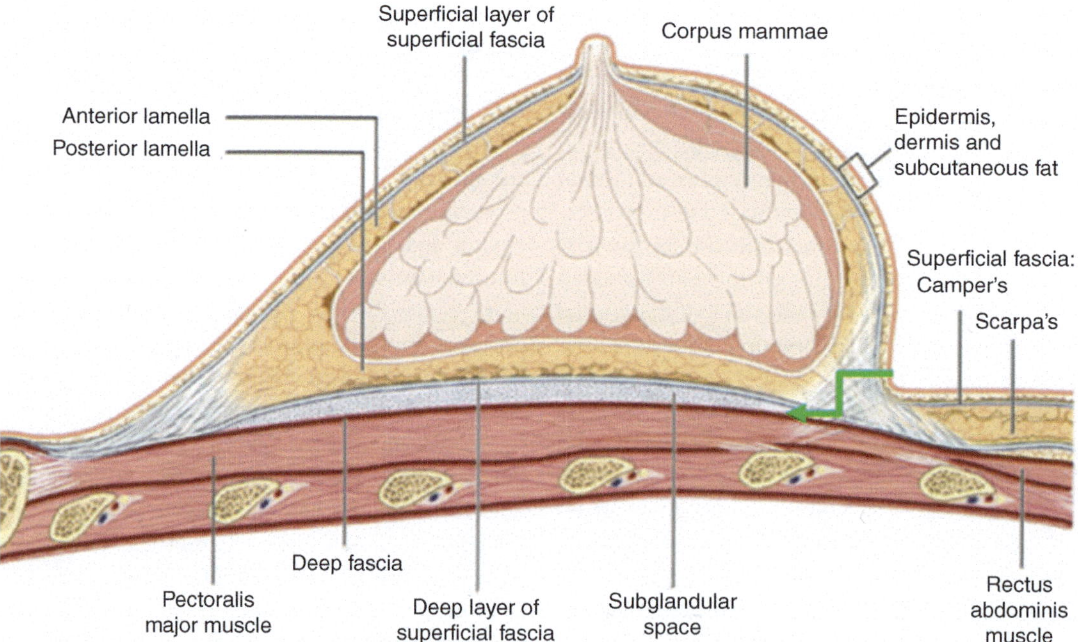

Fig. 1.41 If subfascial pocket with lowering of the IMF is intended, the native IMF must be disrupted to minimize the risk of double-bubble deformity. The course of dissection from the new site of IMF to the subfascial pocket is depicted in green arrow. (Modified and used with permission. Copyright © Susan Gilbert)

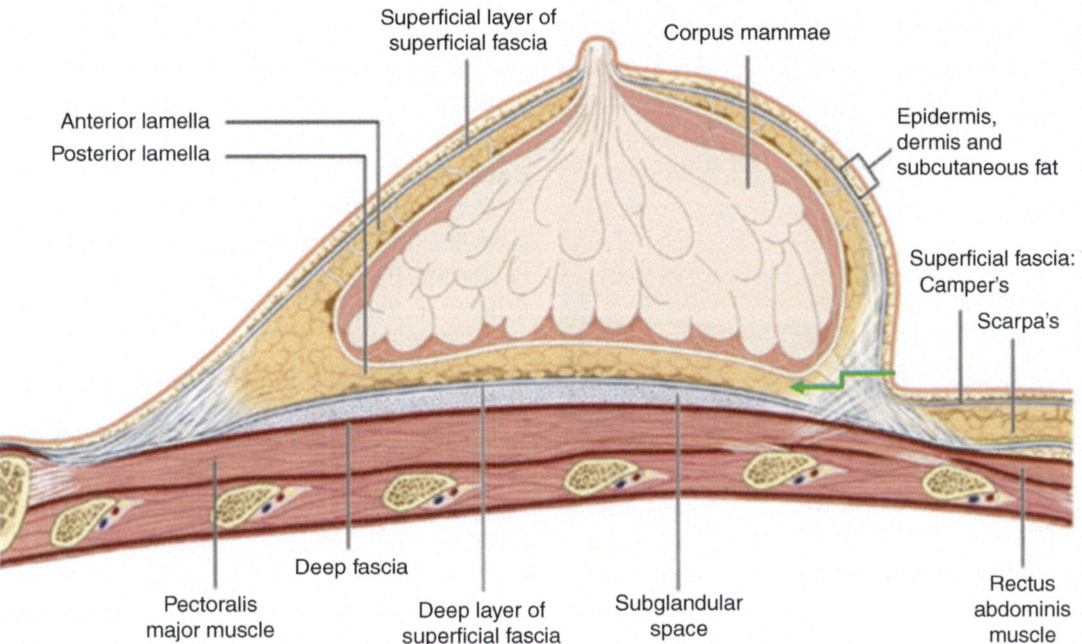

Fig. 1.42 If subglandular pocket with lowering of the IMF is intended, the native IMF must be disrupted to minimize the risk of double-bubble deformity. The course of dissection from the new site of IMF to the subglandular pocket is depicted in green arrow. (Modified and used with permission. Copyright © Susan Gilbert)

Furthermore, meticulous care should be taken to make the surgery bloodless.

Postoperative Care

The patient is discharged and seen in the office the following morning. This allows for a review of the postoperative timeline points. The patient is instructed how to perform two simple exercises: bringing the hands together behind the back and then stretching the arms by externally rotating the arms while squeezing shoulder blades together. Both of these exercises stretch the pectoralis major muscle and help reduce pain. If smooth implants are used, we recommend wearing a supportive bra continuously for 6 months in order to reduce the risk of lateral or inferior malposition. This is contraindicated in the case of textured implants as they heal where they are placed and wearing bras may displace them superiorly (Fig. 1.43).

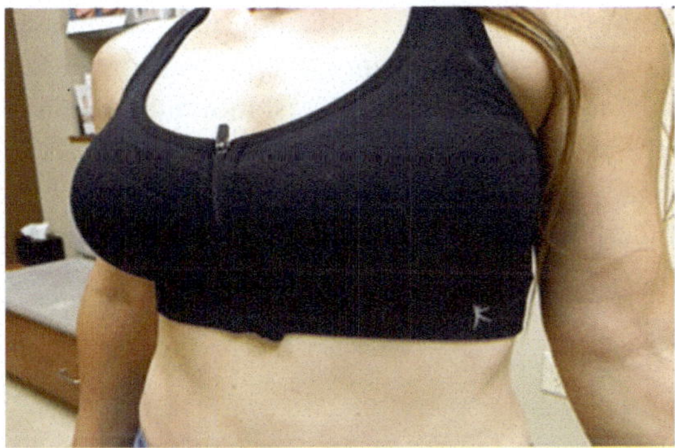

Fig. 1.43 Supportive postoperative bra for breast augmentation with smooth round implants

Postoperatively, if the lower pole is still tight after a couple of weeks, the surgeon can consider the upper pole elastic band to encourage lower pole stretching (Fig. 1.44).

For the first 3 weeks, the range of motion for the arms is limited to 90° at the shoulders in order to protect the IMF fixation. After 3 weeks, patient is allowed to use the arms in full range

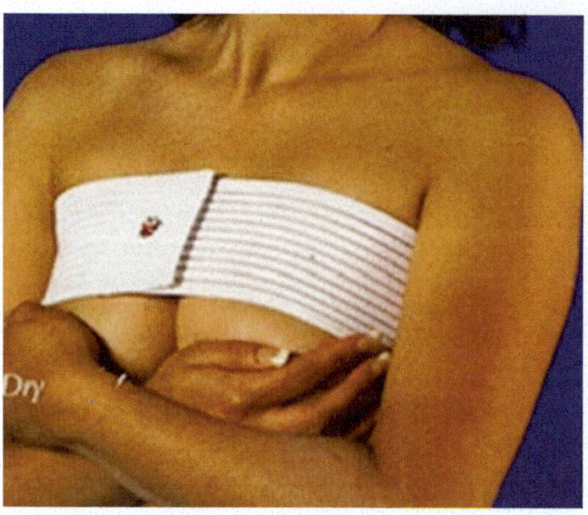

Fig. 1.44 Upper pole compression garment can help with stretching of a very tight lower pole postoperatively

of motion. Patient is also not allowed to engage in any strenuous activities for the first 6 weeks while the capsule is maturing [40]. At 3 weeks, the patient returns for a postoperative visit, at which time she is given the scar product. At 6-month follow-up, the patient comes back to discuss the postoperative result. This provides the opportunity to remind the patient about the importance of self-examination, the recommendation regarding implant surveillance (with either non-contrast MRI or high-resolution ultrasound) to assess its integrity and a reminder about BIA-ALCL. Patients are encouraged to return every other year. It is also important to take postoperative photographs of their breasts at each visit, which can serve as a good reference should any changes happen.

Case Presentations

Case 1

A 45-year-old g2p1 who underwent bilateral augmentation with smooth round full profile gel implants (Allergan, SSF), size 295 cc on the right and 265 cc on the left with 2-year follow-up. Note good lateral pocket stability in prone position (Fig. 1.45).

Case 2

A 38-year-old g2p2 with postpartum breast atrophy, grade II ptosis, and abdominal laxity, who underwent bilateral DP2 submuscular breast augmentation with smooth round full profile gel implants (Allergan SSF), size 385 cc along with periareolar mastopexy and high lateral tension abdominoplasty with 2-year follow-up (Fig. 1.46).

Case 3

A 35-year-old g2p2 with postpartum breast atrophy with constricted bases and short lower poles, who underwent bilateral DP2 submuscular breast augmentation with textured high-profile tear-shaped gel implants with short height and size 385 cc with 2-year follow-up. She required lowering of the IMFs and radial release in order to expand the lower pole. The IMF incision is where the new IMF is. Note the improvement in nipple symmetry due to the higher profile implant in the lower pole expanding the lower pole (controlled tissue expansion) and pushing the NAC upward (Fig. 1.47).

Case 4

A 36-year-old g3p3 postpartum breast atrophy,who underwent bilateral subfascial breast augmentation using textured high-profile tear-shaped gel implants with short height and size 370 cc on the right and 325 cc on the left side with 2-year follow-up. Patient desired a more natural look without disruption of the pectoralis function (Fig. 1.48).

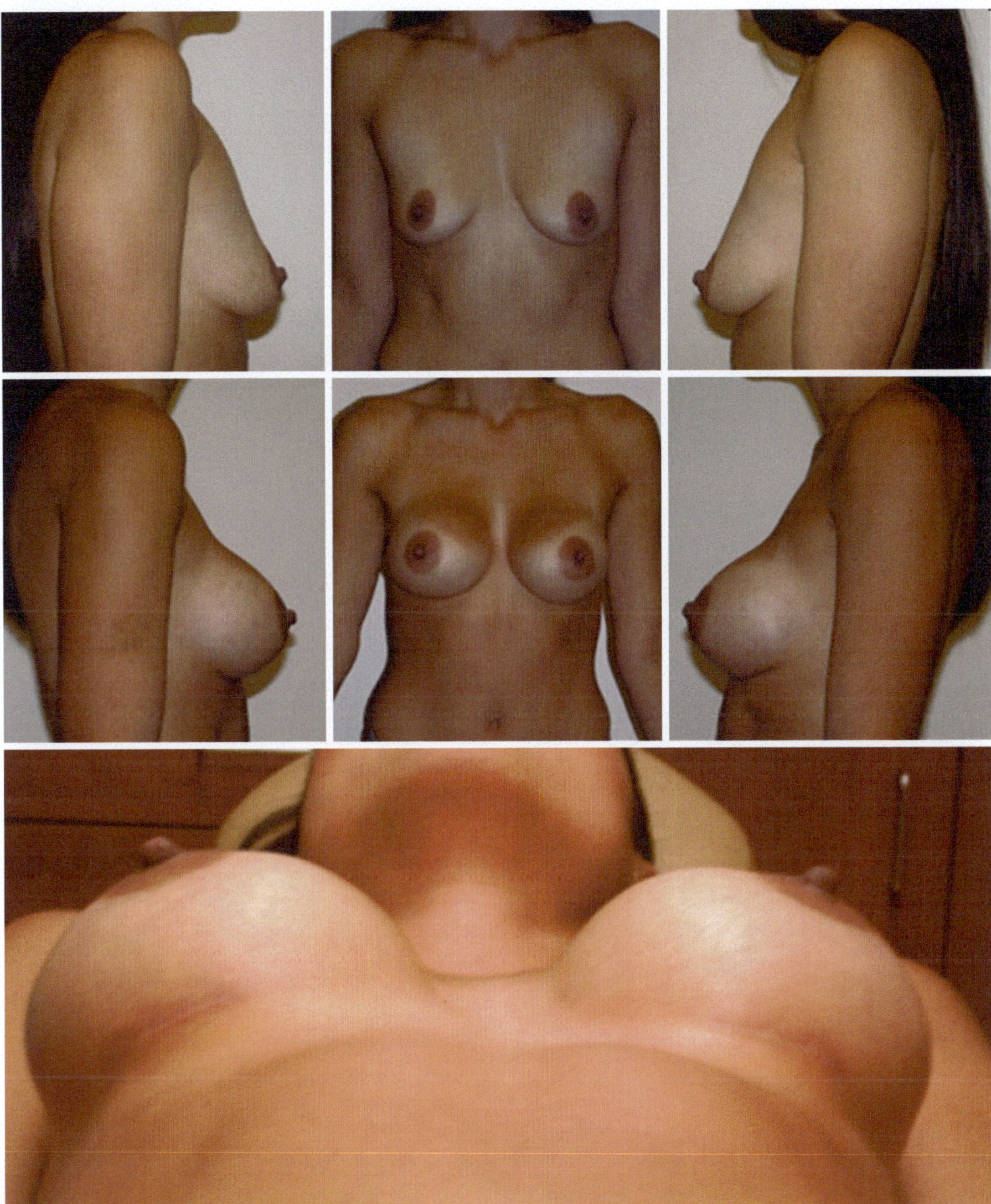

Fig. 1.45 Case 1

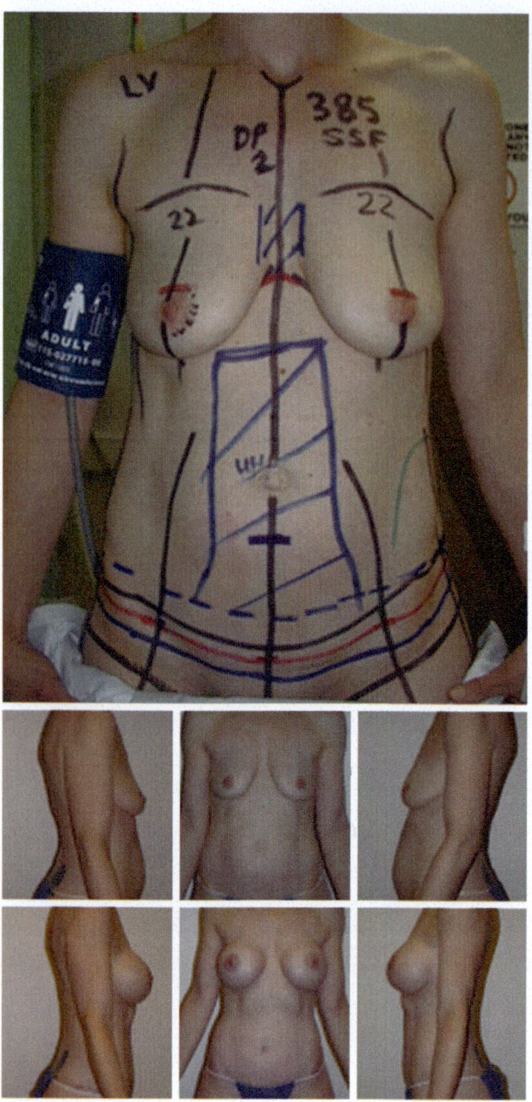

Fig. 1.46 Case 2

Case 5

A 28-year-old g0p0 who underwent bilateral breast augmentation in DP1 using smooth round moderate plus profile gel implants (Mentor, MPP) and size 255 cc with 3-year follow-up (Fig. 1.49).

Case 6

A 26-year-old G0P0 who underwent bilateral submuscular breast augmentation in DP1 with moderated plus profile smooth round saline implants (Mentor, MPP), size 275 cc filled to 300 cc with 2-year follow-up (Fig. 1.50).

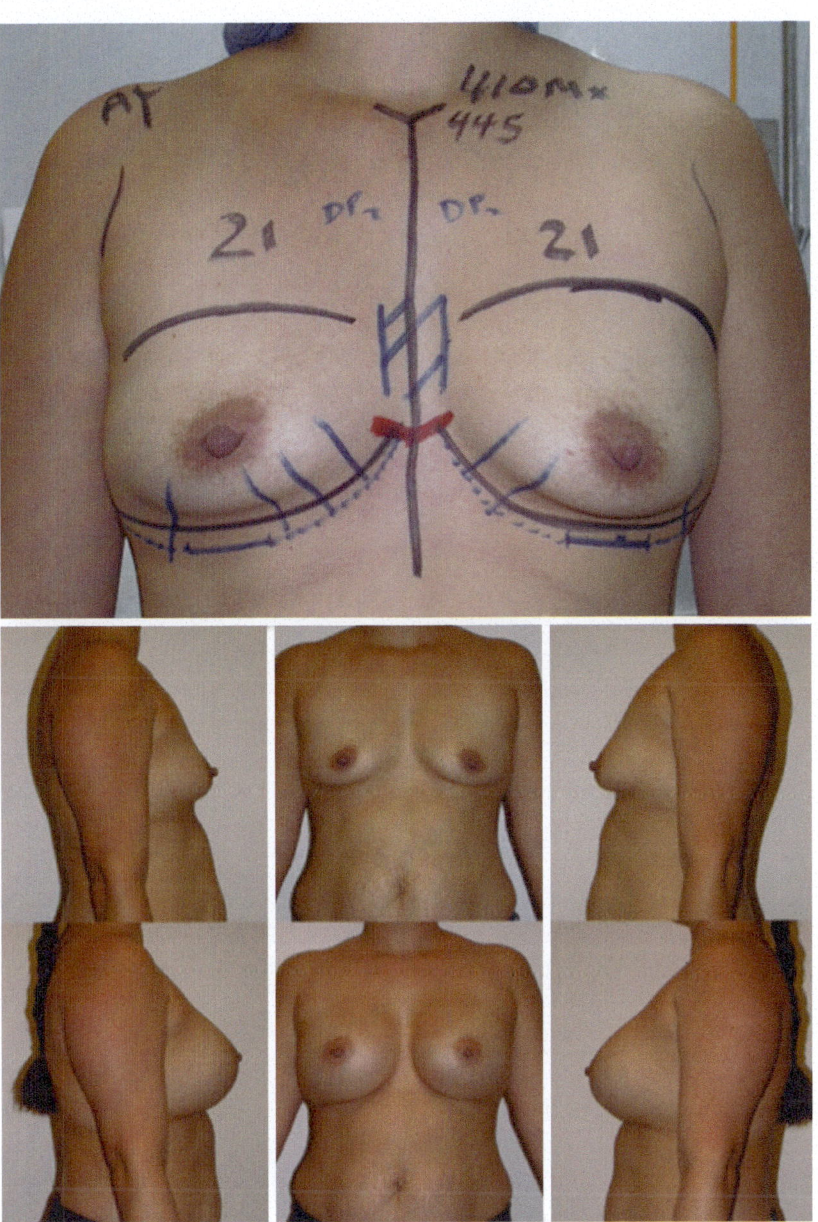

Fig. 1.47 Case 3

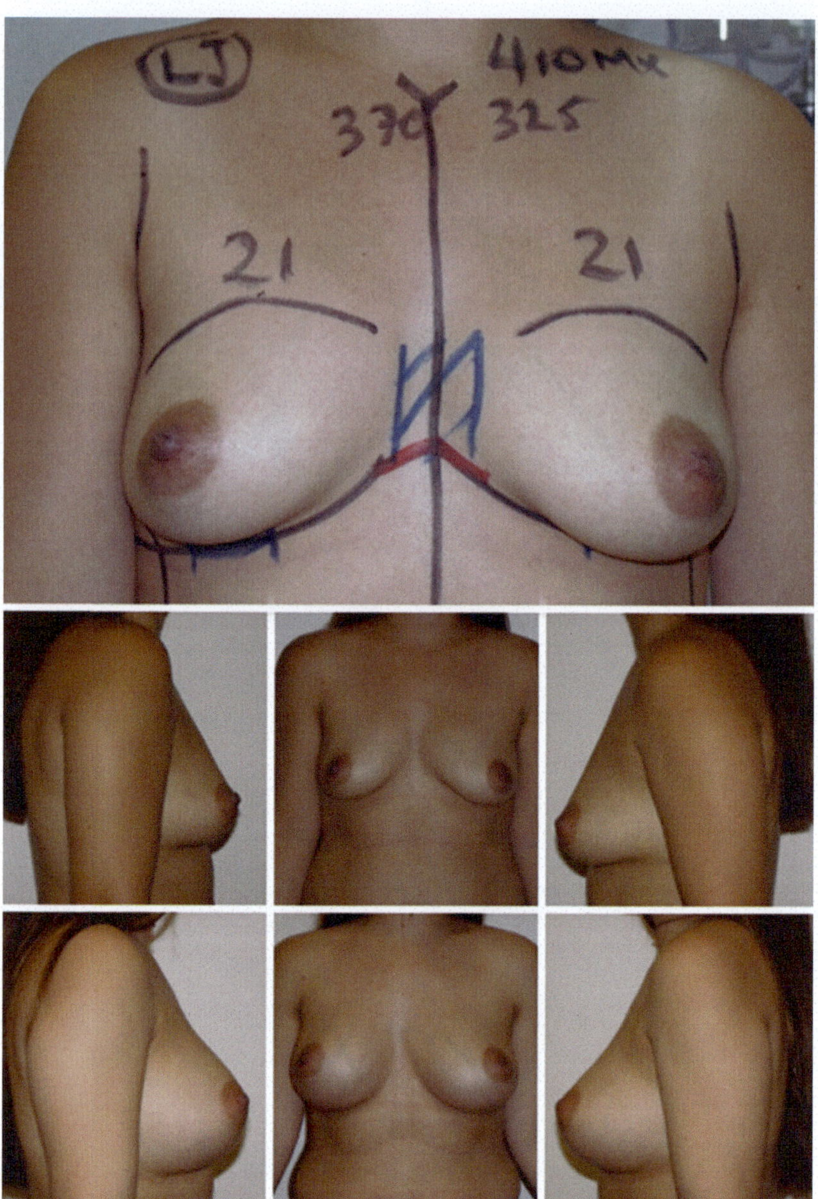

Fig. 1.48 Case 4

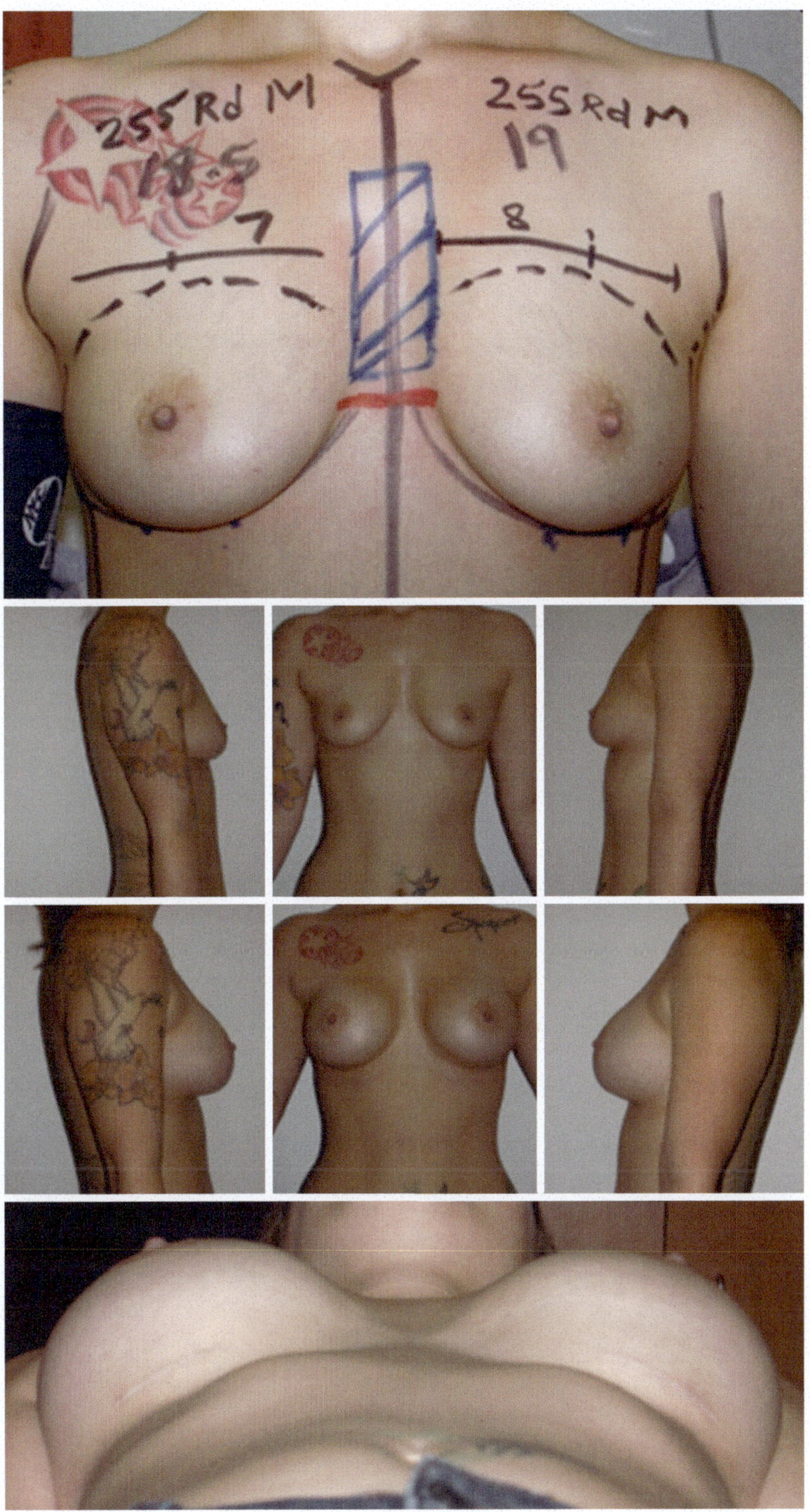

Fig. 1.49 Case 5

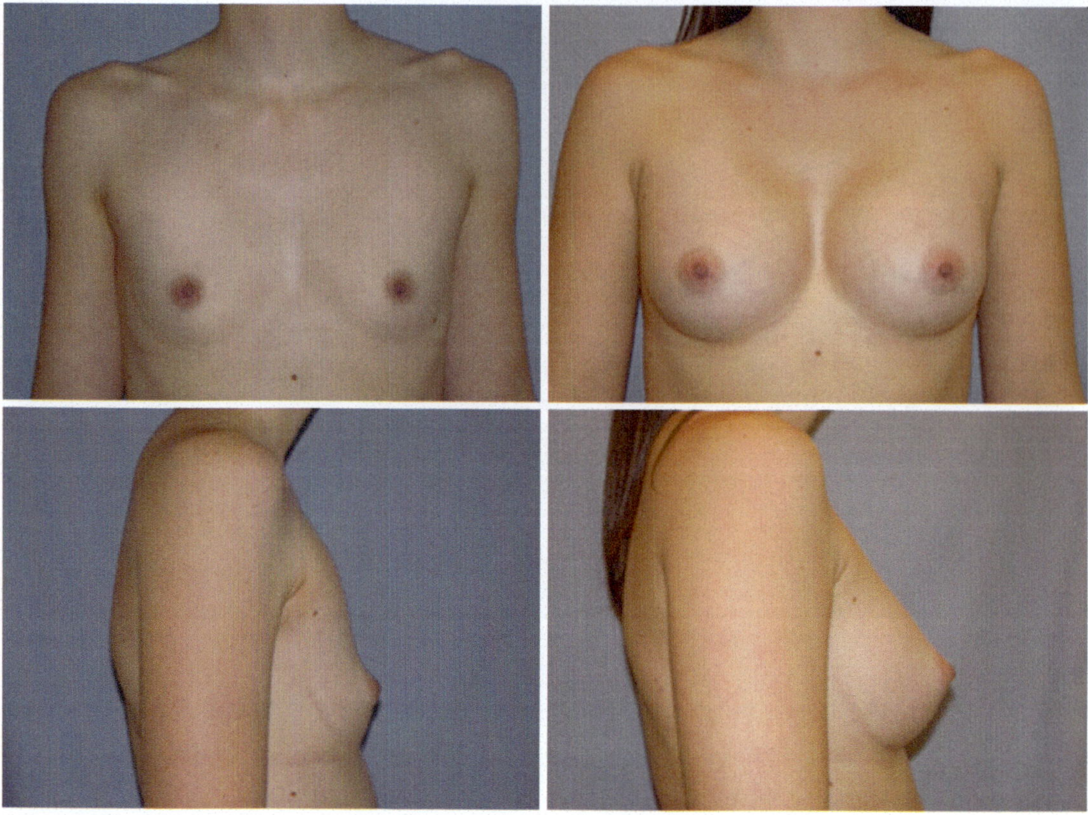

Fig. 1.50 Case 6

Conclusion

Breast augmentation with implants continues to evolve with the goal of improving surgical and aesthetic outcomes. The ability to successfully augment a breast with prosthetic devices depends on the surgeon's ability to follow certain principles of proper patient selection, proper implant selection based on biodimensional planning, and meticulous surgical execution. The strict adherence to these principles leads to a result that is predictable, reliable, and highly satisfying with less risk of reoperation.

Clinical Caveats

- The inframammary incisions determine the new IMF location. They should be placed based on the implant width (*X*) with textured implants requiring a longer N:IMF distance than the smooth implants.
- The circummammary ligament is weaker laterally. The width of the pocket is the width of the implant (*X*) not the breast; Do NOT over dissect especially with smooth implants to reduce the risk of malposition. Over dissection of the pocket medially increases the risk of symmastia and disruption of the origin of the muscle.
- Large implants, that is, implants greater than 400 cc, tend to have higher complication rates. Remind the patient that sometimes the short-term satisfaction is not compatible with long-term durability.
- IMF incision is the preferred location in order to minimize exposure to the bacteria in breast parenchyma.

- The "no touch" technique is used to reduce biofilm exposure.
- If prepectoral pocket is chosen, the subfascial plane is preferred to minimize potential biofilm exposure from breast parenchyma and preserve the Cooper's ligaments.
- If IMF lowering is indicated, one must release the IMF in the proper plane in accordance to the pocket location in order to avoid double-bubble deformity.

References

1. 2018 Cosmetic (Aesthetic) Surgery National Data Bank. The American Society for Aesthetic Plastic Surgery. https://www.surgery.org/sites/default/files/ASAPS-Stats2018.pdf.
2. Dickinson BP, Handel N. Approaching revisional surgery in augmentation and mastopexy/augmentation patients. Ann Plast Surg. 2012;68:12–6.
3. Suri S, Bagiella E, Factor S, Taub P. Soft tissue adjuncts in revisionary breast revisionary aesthetic surgery. Ann Plast Surg. 2107;78:230–5.
4. Brown MH, Somogyi RB, Aggarwal S. Secondary breast augmentation. Plast Reconstr Surg. 2016;138:119e.
5. Patrick Maxwell PG, Gabriel A. Acellular dermal matrix for reoperative breast augmentation. Plast Reconstr Surg. 2014;134:932.
6. Types of Breast Implants. FDA U.S. Food and Drug Administration. Oct 2019. https://www.fda.gov/medical-devices/breast-implants/types-breast-implants.
7. Blackburn VF, Blackburn AV. Taking a history in aesthetic surgery: SAGA--the surgeon's tool for patient selection. J Plast Reconstr Aesthet Surg. 2008;61:723–9.
8. Crerand CE, Franklin ME, Sarwer DB. Body dysmorphic disorder and cosmetic surgery. Plast Reconstr Surg. 2006;118:167e–80e.
9. Sarwer DB. The psychological aspects of cosmetic breast augmentation. Plast Reconstr Surg. 2007;120:110S–7S.
10. Stevens WG, Pacella SJ, Gear AJ, Freeman ME, McWhorter C, Tenenbaum MJ, et al. Clinical experience with a fourth-generation textured silicone gel breast implant: a review of 1012 Mentor MemoryGel breast implants. Aesthet Surg J. 2008;28:642–7.
11. Spear SL, Heden P. Allergan's silicone gel breast implants. Expert Rev Med Devices. 2007;4:699–708.
12. Cash TF, Duel LA, Perkins LL. Women's psychosocial outcomes of breast augmentation with silicone gel-filled implants: a 2-year prospective study. Plast Reconstr Surg. 2002;109:2112–21; discussion 2122–2113.
13. Solvi AS, Foss K, von Soest T, Roald HE, Skolleborg KC, Holte A. Motivational factors and psychological processes in cosmetic breast augmentation surgery. J Plast Reconstr Aesthet Surg. 2010;63(4):673–80.
14. Tebbetts JB. Achieving a predictable 24-hour return to normal activities after breast augmentation: part II. Patient preparation, refined surgical techniques, and instrumentation. Plast Reconstr Surg. 2002;109:293–305; discussion 306–297.
15. Clemens MW, Jacobsen ED, Horwitz SM. 2019 NCCN consensus guidelines on the diagnosis and treatment of breast implant-associated anaplastic large cell lymphoma (BIA-ALCL). Aesthet Surg J. 2019;39(S1):S3–S13.
16. Coroneos CJ, Selber JC, Offodile AC, Butler CE, Clemens MW. US FDA breast implant postapproval studies: long-term outcomes in 99,993 patients. Ann Surg. 2019;269(1):30–6.
17. Sieber DA, Adams WP. What's your micromort? A patient-oriented analysis of breast implant-associated anaplastic large cell lymphoma (BIA-ALCL). Aesthet Surg J. 2017;37(8):887–91.
18. FDA Update on the Safety of Silicone Gel-Filled Breast Implants. Center for Devices and Radiological Health U.S. Food and Drug Administration. June 2011. https://www.fda.gov/media/80685/download.
19. Abernethy A, Shuren J. Statement on the agency's continued efforts to project women's health and enhance safety information available to patients considering breast implants. FDA U.S. Food and Drug Administration. Oct 2019. https://www.fda.gov/news-events/press-announcements/statement-agencys-continued-efforts-protect-womens-health-and-enhance-safety-information-available.
20. Tebbetts JB. Dual plane breast augmentation: optimizing implant-soft-tissue relationships in a wide range of breast types. Plast Reconstr Surg. 2001;107:1255–72.
21. Derby BM, Codner MA. Textured silicone breast implant use in primary augmentation: Core data update and review. Plast Reconstr Surg. 2015;135:113.
22. Montenmurro P, Cheema M, Hedén P, Ferri M, Quattrini Li A, Avvedimento S. Role of macro-textured shaped extra full projection cohesive gel implants in primary breast augmentation. Aesthet Surg J. 2017;37(4):408–18.
23. Hall-Findlay EJ. The three breast dimensions: analysis and effecting change. Plast Reconstr Surg. 2010;125:1632.
24. Tebbetts JB, Adams WP. Five critical decisions in breast augmentation using five measurements in 5 minutes: the high five decision support process. Plast Reconstr Surg. 2005;116:2005–16.
25. Adams WP Jr. The process of breast augmentation: four sequential steps for optimizing outcomes for patients. Plast Reconstr Surg. 2008;122:1892–900.

26. Lee MR, Unger JG, Adams WP Jr. The tissue-based triad: a process approach to augmentation mastopexy. Plast Reconstr Surg. 2014;134:215.
27. Adams WP Jr, Mckee D. Matching the implant to the breast: a systematic review of implant size selection systems for breast augmentation. Plast Reconstr Surg. 2016;138:987.
28. Kortesis BG, Bharti G. Maximizing aesthetics and patient selection utilizing Natrelle Inspira line implants in aesthetic breast surgery. Plast Reconstr Surg. 2019;144:30S.
29. Calobrace BM, Stevens WG, Capizzi PJ, Cohen R, et al. Risk factor analysis for capsular contracture: a 10-year Sientra study using round, smooth, and textured implants for breast augmentation. Plast Reconstr Surg. 2018;141:20S.
30. Araco A, Caruso R, Araco F, Overton J, Gravante G. Capsular contractures: a systematic review. Plast Reconstr Surg. 2009;124(6):1808–19.
31. Wong CH, Samuel M, Tan BK, Song C. Capsular contracture in subglandular breast augmentation with textured versus smooth breast implants: a systematic review. Plast Reconstr Surg. 2006;118(5):1224–36.
32. Dinah W, Rohrich RJ. The management of capsular contracture in breast augmentation: a systematic review. Plast Reconstr Surg. 2016;137:826.
33. Stevens WG, Nahabedian MY, Calobrace B, Harrington JL, Capizzi PJ, Cohen R, et al. Five-year analysis for capsular contracture: a 5-year Sientra study analysis using round, smooth, and textured implants for breast augmentation. Plast Reconstr Surg. 2013;132:1115.
34. Lesavoy MA, Trussler AP, Dickinson BP. Difficulties with subpectoral augmentation mammaplasty and its correction: the role of subglandular site change in revision aesthetic breast surgery. Plast Reconstr Surg. 2010;125:363.
35. Rehnke RD, Groening RM, Van Buskirk ER, Clarke JM. Anatomy of the superficial fascia system of the breast: a comprehensive theory of breast fascial anatomy. Plast Reconstr Surg. 2018;142:1135.
36. Galdiero M, Larocca F, Iovene MR, et al. Microbial evaluation in capsular contracture of breast implants. Plast Reconstr Surg. 2018;141:23.
37. Randquist C, Gribbe Ö. Highly cohesive textured form stable gel implants: principles and technique. Chapter 23. In: Aesthetic and reconstructive surgery of the breast. Philadelphia: Saunders; 2010. p. 339–55.
38. Graf RM, Bernardes A, Rippel R, Araujo LR, Damasio RC, Auersvald A. Subfascial breast implant: a new procedure. Plast Reconstr Surg. 2003;111:904–8.
39. Siclovan HR, Jomah JA. Advantages and outcomes in subfascial breast augmentation: a two-year review of experience. Aesthet Plast Surg. 2008;32:426–31.
40. Kronowitz SJ. Delayed-immediate breast reconstruction: technical and timing considerations. Plast Reconstr Surg. 2010;125:463–74.

Shaping the Breast: Augmentation Mastopexy

2

M. Bradley Calobrace and Chet Mays

Introduction

Breast ptosis is one of the most common problems encountered by plastic surgeons. Although it can be developmental in nature, it is more commonly acquired secondary to weight loss, hormonal changes, pregnancy, and/or aging. When considering which surgical approach will be employed to "shape" the breast, the physical characteristics of the breast and the patient's desired aesthetic outcome must be considered. When evaluating the ptotic breast, the volume status of the breasts should be a part of the initial assessment. A mastopexy alone is reserved for a patient in whom the major concern is breast ptosis and not an issue of breast volume or upper pole fullness, as the procedure repositions the breast with only limited removal or transposition of breast tissue. Patients with volume deficiencies or desiring significant upper pole volume require placement of an implant with the mastopexy to achieve their desired shape.

To achieve these objectives, the breast augmentation and the mastopexy be performed either simultaneous or as a staged procedure. Much controversy has existed over the years as to the safety of doing this procedure as one-stage [1–3]. Distractors believe a two-stage procedure produces superior aesthetic results and is a much safer approach compared to a one-stage procedure. However, significant data and reports have emerged over the past few years demonstrating the safety and efficacy of these procedures being performed simultaneously [4–8].

Careful perioperative decision-making is required to achieve a successful outcome in augmentation mastopexy surgery. The surgical approach to the patient with ptotic breast desiring and/or requiring a breast implant for correction is determined following a thorough evaluation. This evaluation should include appropriate breast measurements, breast tissue density, quality of skin, NAC (nipple–areolar complex) and breast ptosis, chest wall characteristics, breast footprint, and the patient's expectations in planning for the procedure. For the patient with limited ptosis, a breast augmentation alone may provide adequate rejuvenation. If a mastopexy is deemed necessary with the augmentation, many types of mastopexy techniques described to address the ptotic breast can be utilized, including circumareolar, circumvertical, circumvertical with IMF wedge, inframammary technique, or the inverted-T scar

M. B. Calobrace (✉)
CaloAesthetics Plastic Surgery Center, Louisville, KY, USA

University of Louisville Division of Plastic Surgery, Louisville, KY, USA

University of Kentucky Division of Plastic Surgery, Louisville, KY, USA
e-mail: drbrad@calobrace.com

C. Mays
CaloAesthetics Plastic Surgery Center, Louisville, KY, USA

University of Louisville Division of Plastic Surgery, Louisville, KY, USA

K. Movassaghi (ed.), *Shaping the Breast*, https://doi.org/10.1007/978-3-030-59777-1_2

technique [9–13]. It is important to remember that the skin excision design is not the pedicle design for the procedure. Whereas the pedicle refers to the design for blood supply to the NAC, the skin excision design determines the final scar locations and can be based on many different pedicles. An inverted-T design does not need to be an inferior pedicle and can often be used with a superior, medial, or superiomedial pedicle [11].

For a single-stage augmentation mastopexy, the optimal implant pocket must also be determined including dual-plane submuscular, subfascial, or subglandular. The pocket selection impacts the surgical approach, the vascularity of the skin flaps and NAC, and long-term outcome. Likewise, a wide variety of breast implant options are available to optimize results. Implant characteristics including implant fill, shell texturization, silicone gel cohesiveness, gel-to-shell fill ratios, gel–shell interaction, projections, and shape can impact complication rates, as well as the aesthetics of the final result [14, 15].

Of course, the operative approach which is based on all the decisions leading up to the surgery is likewise of immense importance in achieving success. The operative approach should always prioritize safety with an effort not to compromise the final aesthetic result. In this chapter, the details of the surgical technique will be explored with a focus on the use of a variety of mastopexy designs, pockets, implants, and the modifications required in the technique to optimize the outcome with each of the different options available to the surgeon. It is the marriage of decision-making with expert execution that leads to the highest level of safety, optimal aesthetic outcomes, and high patient satisfaction.

Preoperative Evaluation

The evaluation should begin with a breast exam with breast measurements including the base width, sternal notch to nipple distance, nipple to fold distance (at rest and under maximal stretch), and assessment of thickness with a pinch test (Fig. 2.1).

The amount of ptosis present should also be assessed. Ptosis has classically been described as per Regnault based on the relationship of the NAC to the inframammary fold [16]. Although

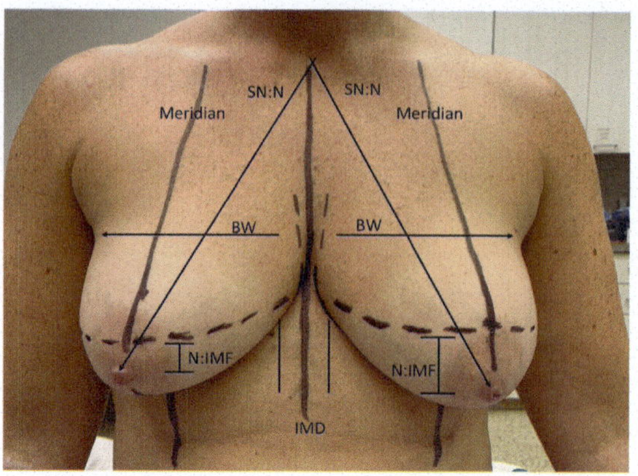

Fig. 2.1 Breast measurements: sternal notch to nipple, SN:N; breast width, BW; nipple to inframammary fold distance, N:IMF; intermammary distance, IMD. The dotted line represents the transposed inframammary fold

this provides some information about the degree of breast ptosis, it in of itself is insufficient to describe the true extent of breast ptosis.

Patients with different grades of ptosis per the Regnault's classification may have completely different breast compositions including the quality of breast tissue and skin, the quantity of breast tissue present, and the vertical excess present as shown in Fig. 2.2.

A more complete assessment of ptosis is summarized in Table 2.1.

Assessment should also include evaluation of the skin thickness and elasticity, the quantity and distribution of subcutaneous fat, the composition and firmness of the breast parenchyma, the integrity of the Cooper's ligaments, the nature and position of the underlying musculature, and the shape and slope of the underlying chest wall. All these aspects of the breast composition influence the shape of the breast and ultimately the outcome after the augmentation mastopexy.

Determining the amount of vertical excess that is present will assist in determining the type of mastopexy should be accomplished. It also can assist in determining the appropriate patients for staging [7]. Patients with similar levels of ptosis can have quite different amounts of vertical excess as was shown in Fig. 2.2. To determine the vertical excess (VE), the new nipple position distance to the new inframammary fold is subtracted from the new nipple position and the patient's actual inframammary fold (Table 2.2). The "new IMF" is determined by selecting the new nipple position, then adding 2 cm

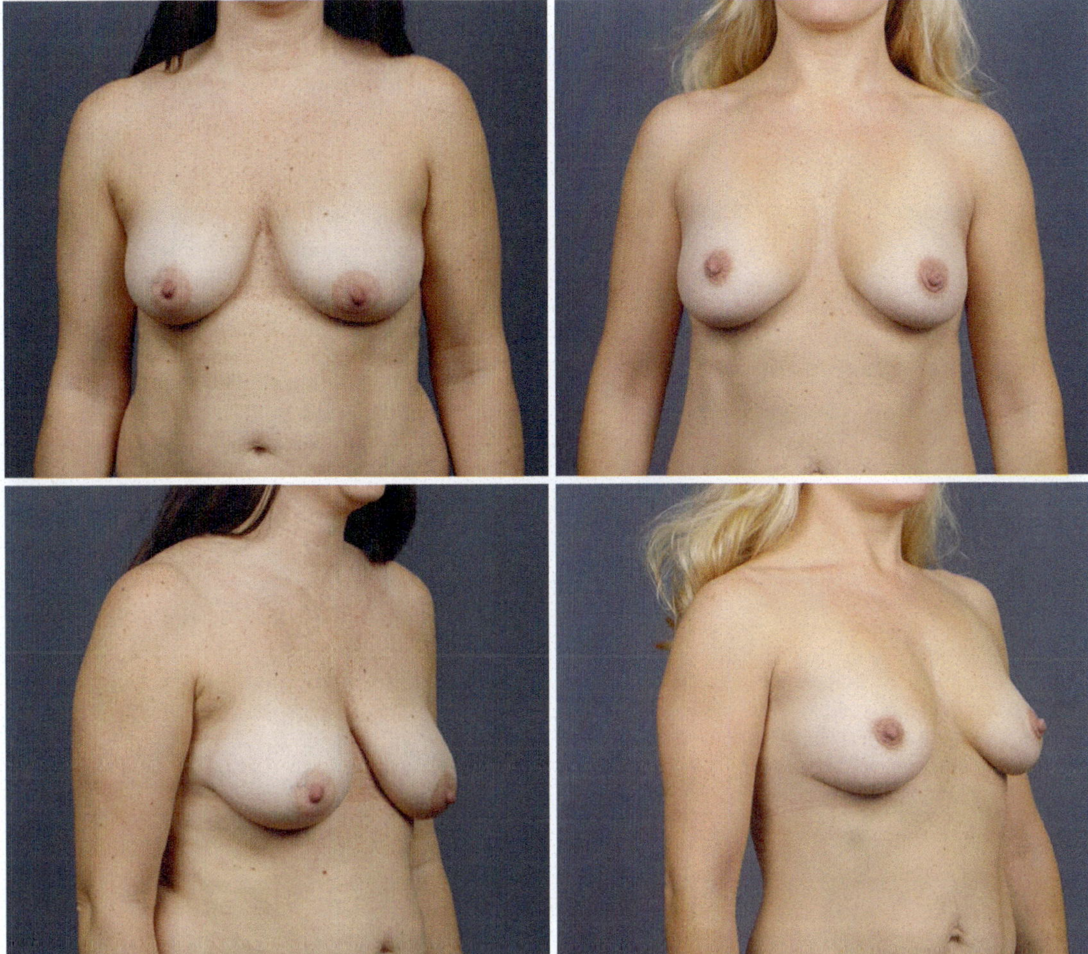

Fig. 2.2 Two patients shown with Grade I ptosis where the nipple is at the IMF. The patient on the right side has greater vertical excess from the nipple to IMF position

Table 2.1 Assessment of breast ptosis

Relationship of the NAC to the IMF (Regnault's degree of ptosis)
Grade 1: nipple at the level of the inframammary fold, above the lower contour of the gland
Grade 2: nipple below the level of the inframammary fold, above the lower contour of the gland
Grade 3: nipple below the level of the inframammary fold, at the lower contour of the gland
Amount of breast tissue overhanging the fold
Location of the NAC on the breast mound
Amount of vertical excess and horizontal excess
Footprint of the breast on the chest wall – low, medium, high
Quality and quantity of breast parenchyma and skin

for ½ the areola diameter and an additional 6–8 cm for the lower pole skin that will be required for the new breast shape. Thus, it is almost always 8–10 cm inferior to the new identified nipple position. This lower pole arc length is estimated based on the final breast size, which will include the implant and the native breast tissue. This is true for mastopexies, breast reductions, and augmentation mastopexies. All of the additional skin present from the "new IMF" to the original IMF is the vertical excess (Fig. 2.3). When the vertical excess is greater than 8–10 cm, a staged augmentation mastopexy should be considered (Fig. 2.4).

Table 2.2 Vertical excess

Vertical excess (VE)
VE = New Nipple to actual IMF – New N to new IMF
VE > 8–10 cm consider staging augmentation mastopexy

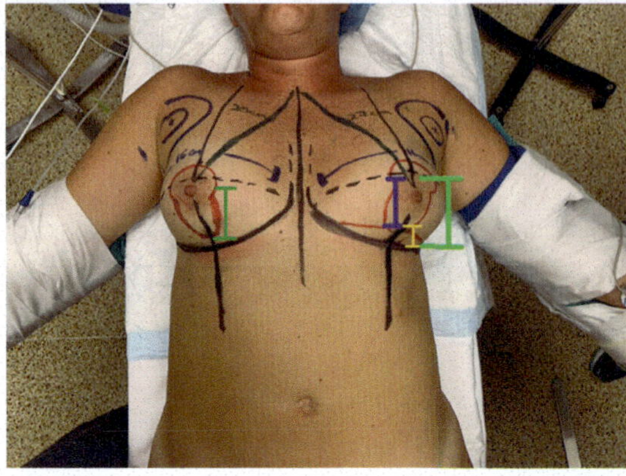

Fig. 2.3 Vertical excess (yellow line) shown on the left breast represents the new nipple position distance to the new inframammary fold (purple line) subtracted from the new nipple position and the patient's actual Inframammary fold (green line). The right breast in this patient has no vertical excess because the new nipple position to actual fold (green line) is the same as the new nipple to new fold on the left breast

Blood Supply

When performing an augmentation mastopexy, an understanding and assessment of the vascular anatomy is critical to performing the procedure safely. The breast has a rich blood supply from multiple sources, including the internal mammary artery perforators, the lateral thoracic arteries, the thoracoacromial arteries, and the anterolateral and anteromedial intercostal perforators [17].

To insure the most reliable blood supply to the NAC and skin flaps in an augmentation mastopexy, the superior pedicle and occasionally the superomedial pedicles are utilized (Figs. 2.5 and 2.6). The superior pedicle is supplied by the second branch of the internal mammary artery (IMA) that emerges deep from the second interspace and courses superficial across the medial upper breast to enter the NAC slightly medial to the midline and approximately 1 cm deep. The medial pedicle is supplied by the third branch of the IMA that emerges from the third interspace and similarly courses superficially across the breast parenchyma to the medial aspect of the NAC. The superficial position of these vessels in the upper pole allows the implant place-

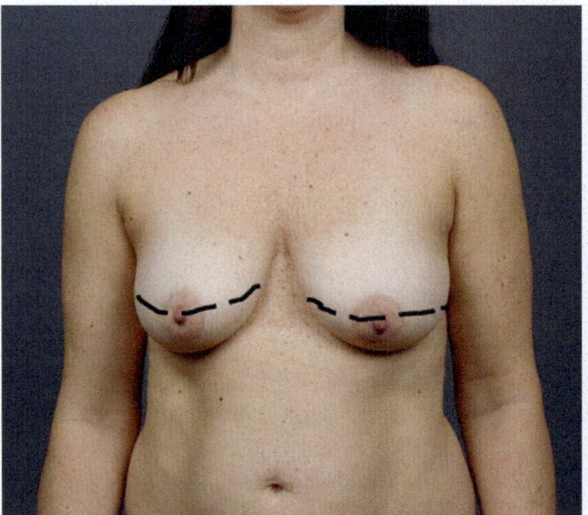

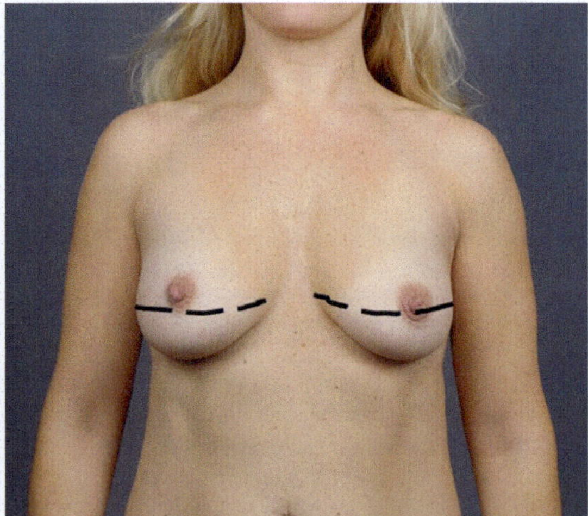

Fig. 2.4 Comparing patients with grade I ptosis but varying degrees of vertical excess. The dotted line represents the transposed IMF

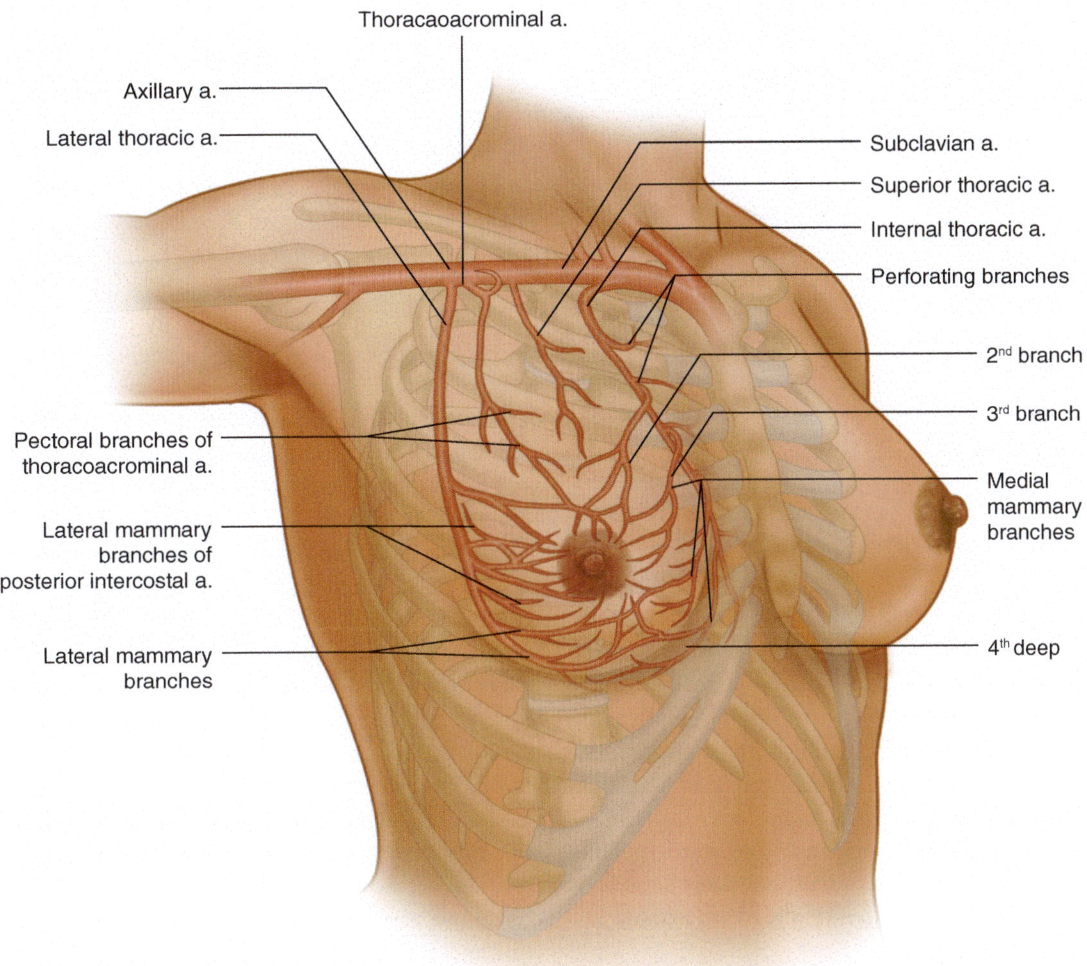

Fig. 2.5 Breast blood supply. The second branch of the internal mammary artery (IMA) supplying the superior pedicle. The third branch of the IMA supplying the medial pedicle. The fourth branch of the IMA supplying the inferior pedicle

ment and mastopexy without interfering with the blood supply.

However, these vessels take origin along the sternal border in the medial aspect of the implant pocket and can be inadvertently sacrificed when aggressive medial pectoral muscle division is performed.

The inferior pedicle is not utilized in an augmentation mastopexy as its blood supply through the deep 4th branch of the IMA is sacrificed with development of the implant pocket and its secondary blood supply along the inframammary fold is divided with the mastopexy.

Thus, an augmentation mastopexy with an inferior pedicle design is not truly supplied by pedicle blood supply in most cases, and the best one can hope for is random blood supply. If the remainder of the mastopexy is performed divid-

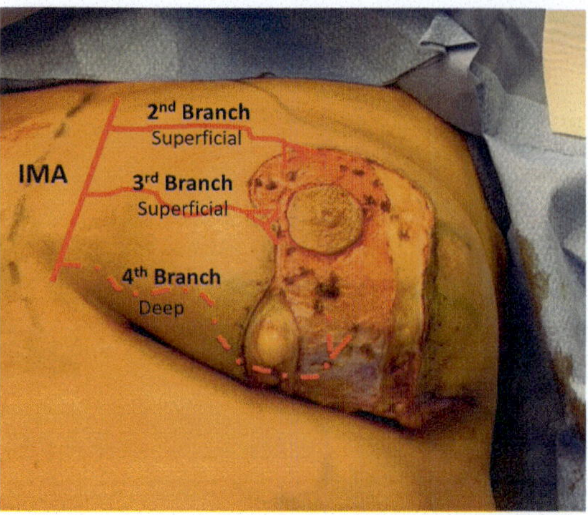

Fig. 2.6 Blood supply to the nipple–areolar complex. The second branch of the internal mammary artery (IMA) supplies the superior pedicle. The third branch of the IMA supplies the medial pedicle. The fourth branch of the IMA running in the deeper plane of the inferior breast is shown with the dotted lines

ing deep into the flaps with an assumption that the inferior pedicle will provide circulation, the division of much needed superficial perforators both medially and laterally can lead to devastating consequences including loss of NAC or breast flap viability and resultant necrosis. Thus, the preferred pedicles enter the breast superiorly and superficially, providing a more reliable and robust blood supply.

Additionally, implant and pocket selection affect the blood supply to the overlying breast. The subpectoral pocket maintains the musculocutaneous perforators (unless an extensive dual plane is performed) and is less likely to interfere with the blood supply compared to a subglandular/subfascial pocket. Likewise, larger implants placed in any pocket, but especially the subglandular/subfascial pocket, may result in undue tension on the mastopexy closure and can create vascular compromise to the NAC or overlying skin flaps, resulting in skin or NAC necrosis.

Patient Expectations

Patients requiring an augmentation mastopexy to shape their breasts have often undergone changes to the breast from weight loss or postpartum and suffer the sequelae of increased laxity of the tissue, stria, nipple and breast ptosis, and loss of parenchymal volume and/or firmness. Patients are often unaware of the challenges faced in their procedure and may be expecting outcomes more in line with a primary breast augmentation. The augmentation mastopexy procedure can be uniquely challenging as it requires enlarging the breast with the augmentation and simultaneously reducing the breast and skin envelope with the mastopexy. Managing expectation in the augmentation mastopexy patient is imperative.

Patients often are unaware of asymmetries, the significant atrophy of the breasts, and differences in the chest wall that affect the final outcome. It is helpful to spend some time determining what shape and outcome the patient would desire, especially in terms of nipple position and volume in the upper pole. The differences in the shape and look that can be achieved with an augmentation mastopexy compared to that of a breast augmentation alone should be discussed. In a recent quality of life study comparing breast augmentation patients to augmentation mastopexy patients, breast augmentation patients were significantly more satisfied with the aesthetic outcome and the quality of life on many psychosocial aspects. The augmentation mastopexy patients reported dissatisfaction with shape, scarring, symmetry, and the nipple–areolar complex [18]. The operative design must consider the patient's desires in an effort to achieve a satisfactory result for the patient. A patient desiring a more natural look may benefit more from a subpectoral implant, a less cohesive implant, or a shaped device, whereas a patient desiring more volume and roundness in the upper pole may require a more cohesive higher profile implant and potentially the implant placed above the muscle. Undoubtedly, there are limitations in what can be achieved in augmentation mastopexy but good perioperative decision-making with an operative approach specifically designed to meet the patient's goals is more likely to provide optimal resulting shape for each patient.

All issues related both to the mastopexy and the augmentation must be discussed including the associated complications and possibly need for revisional procedures. These patients will have scars on the breast, which at times can heal unpredictably, and a clear understanding of the location of the scars and anticipated outcome should be discussed.

Operative Decision-Making

To Stage or Not to Stage

Mastopexy

Correction of breast ptosis may not require both an augmentation and a mastopexy. The ideal candidate for a mastopexy without augmentation is a patient that is relatively satisfied with her volume and is mainly looking for correction in her breast ptosis and improvement in breast shape. The ideal candidate has adequate breast volume and enough ptosis to warrant a mastopexy and the scars associated with these procedures. The patient should be looking for a more natural upper pole, desiring less upper pole convexity and full cleavage. Some patients with ptosis simply need a breast augmentation for improvement.

Augmentation Mastopexy

A patient desiring considerably more volume or significant upper pole volume and cleavage would be better served with an augmentation mastopexy technique. The exception would be the patient desiring those attributes, but the simultaneous procedure is deemed inappropriate or unsafe (Table 2.3). In these cases, a mastopexy can be performed at the initial procedure, followed at least 6 months to 1 year later with a staged breast augmentation (Fig. 2.7).

Table 2.3 Indications for staged augmentation mastopexy

Obesity – BMI >30
Large, pendulous breasts – needs volume reduction
Significant breast ptosis – NAC elevation >5–6 cm
Vertical excess >8–10 cm
Unrealistic expectations – understand reoperation rate >20%
Smokers who refuse to quit

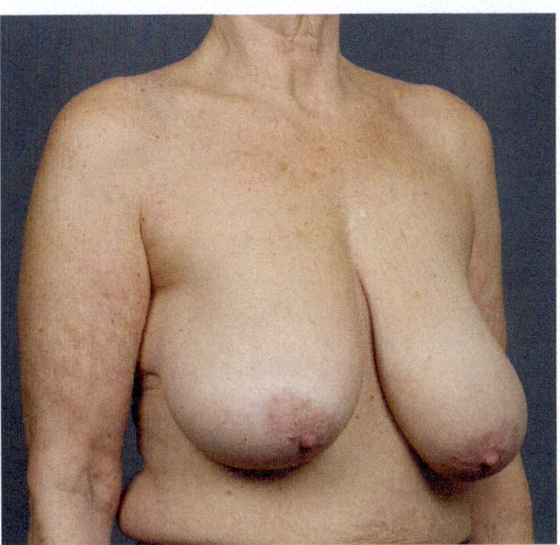

Fig. 2.7 A typical patient who would be a candidate for staging the mastopexy first and then performing the augmentation 6 months to a year later. She has large pendulous breast needing a volume reduction and balancing mastopexy for her grade 3 ptosis

Implant Selection

In augmentation mastopexy, implant selection can significantly impact the final outcome in an augmentation mastopexy case. The implant selection in a one-stage augmentation mastopexy is of greater significance as the augmentation is performed in the face of a mastopexy with soft tissue envelopes which are laxer, stretched, thinned with stria and less tolerant to the effects of the underlying implant.

Implant Profile and Size

Tissue-based planning proves very beneficial in augmentation mastopexy just as it does in augmentation alone [7]. The base width of the breast provides a general guide as to the appropriate sizing of the implant for the breast. In considering implant width, critical to that calculation is determining how much the native breast itself will contribute to the final width of the breast. Optimal implant width is calculated by determining the desired final breast width (usually anterior axillary line to 1 cm from the midline of the chest) minus the soft tissue contribution from the native breast using the medial and lateral pinch:

$$\text{Optimal implant width} = \text{Desired breast width} - \left(1/2\,\text{medial pinch} + 1/2\,\text{Lateral pinch}\right)$$

In a patient with ptosis but with a thin skin brassiere and minimal breast volume, the implant determination will be identical to a straightforward breast augmentation. In breasts with more significant volume and heavier breasts, this calculation might lead to a smaller implant compared to a breast augmentation alone. When trying to achieve a desired volume with limited base width, a higher profile implant may be deemed as appropriate in these patients. However, the skin envelope laxity with the planned mastopexy must be taken into consideration. The effect of a high-profile implant on the skin envelope immediately on the skin flaps and over time with potential for stretch deformity must be balanced against the patient's desire for more volume [19]. In the heavier breasted patient requiring an augmentation and mastopexy, an implant is often selected with a lower profile with greater height and width of the implant to add volume to the upper pole but to minimize the impact on the overlying breast. Oversized implants not only create long term effects, the undue tension created when mastopexy flaps are closed around a larger implant can impact circulation to the NAC and overlying breast skin flaps, leading to ischemia and necrosis. The pocket selection with these implants can also impact circulation. Because of stretch and weight of the implant on the overlying breast tissue, the author prefers silicone implants over saline implants as saline leads to greater lower pole stretch, palpability, visibility, and higher revision rates.

Smooth Versus Textured Implants

Not only the size and profile but also the implant shell that makes up a silicone implant can affect the final outcome. Silicone implants are available as smooth or textured devices. In the United States, smooth implants are utilized in most cases, whereas textured implants predominate in the rest of the world. Smooth implants have several advantages, including a natural mobility and an extremely low risk of wrinkling or palpability. The implants tend to settle at the bottom of the breast pocket and continue to descend with the overlying breast tissue naturally. When performing a mastopexy with the augmentation, the smooth implants can be translocated superiorly taking the tension off the closure and will naturally descend over time back into the newly lifted skin envelope. Due to the laxity of the skin envelopes, surgeons often cite the mobility of the implants as an advantage when there is instability in the overlying breast envelope.

Textured implants have more stability in the breast pocket, whether through implant adherence or simply frictional forces. The more aggressive the texture, in general, the more stable the implant. In the author's opinion, textured implants can significantly improve the quality of results in many augmentation mastopexy patients. The stability imparted seems to create less lower pole stretch deformity over time. Textured implants allow not only for placement of round implants but also for the possibility of using an anatomic-shaped implant. The textured devices, when placed subglandular or subfascial, has been correlated with a lower capsular contracture rate compared to smooth devices [20, 21]. This can liberalize the use of many different pockets in selected patients.

When selecting between a smooth and textured device, the challenge is in trying to determine the optimal implant for each patient while minimizing unwanted sequelae. In the author's experience, textured devices can provide excellent stability in an otherwise unstable breast envelope and is the implant of choice in many patients. Patients with sloping chest walls are also ideal for textured devices as the texture stabilizes the implant and minimizes migration, especially lateral slip of the implant into the axilla. Patients with firm parenchyma and good soft tissue coverage are ideal for a textured implant. When the laxity is too great, as in a weight loss patient, it can be challenging to stabilize the skin envelope adequately over the textured implants. There is an increased risk of waterfall deformity when textured implants are placed under very lax skin

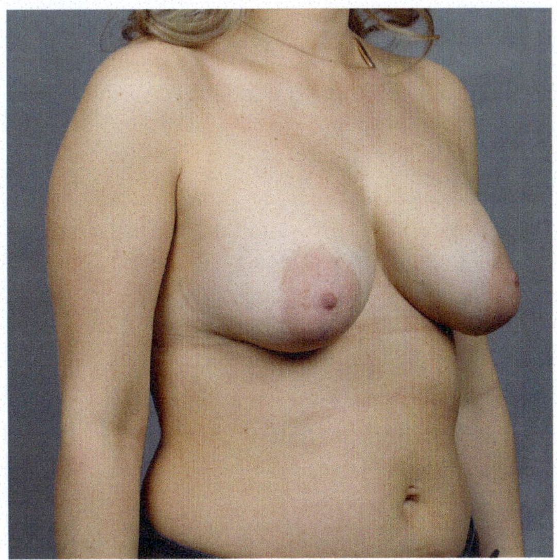

Fig. 2.8 Waterfall deformity

envelopes, and the benefits of stability have to be weighed against this possibility (Fig. 2.8).

Textured implants are more likely to wrinkle compared to a smooth silicone implant. When the skin envelope is thin and wrinkling is a possibility postoperatively, a smooth device may prove advantageous. The newer, more cohesive implants with optimal fills have significantly decreased the amount of wrinkling seen, thus the difference between smooth and textured as it relates to wrinkling may be more theoretical than reality. Textured devices have additional concerns, including double capsule formation, late seromas, and the emerging relationship to BIA-ALCL (breast implant associated-anaplastic large cell lymphoma) [22–24]. The advantages of the textured device in any clinical situation must therefore be weighed against the possibilities of these unfortunate sequelae and the possibilities discussed openly and frankly as part of the consent process.

Shaped Implants

Shaped implants can provide advantages in certain types of patients and may be appropriate in an augmentation mastopexy. Of course, all shaped implants are textured, so the advantages and disadvantages of textured devices apply when considering a shaped device.

There are many varieties of shaped devices, and all the manufacturers have a matrix of choices available to accommodate different shaped breasts and chest walls. Shaped implants in general create a more natural sloping upper pole. Due to the increased cohesiveness of the gel, however, the upper pole volume may be more stable compared to other implants. An implant that is taller than it is wide can provide a nice volume distribution for a long-chested patient with a low breast footprint without over-augmenting the breast. A patient with a high footprint or a very wide base width can benefit from a shaped implant that is wider than it is tall, allowing improved cleavage without over-augmenting the breast and/or upper poles of the breast.

Shaped implants are uniquely beneficial when performing an augmentation mastopexy on patients with constricted breast or tuberous breast deformities. These augmentations are often performed in conjunction with a circumareolar mastopexy to optimize results. The shaped implant provides a point of maximal projection lower than a round implant allowing improved expansion and nipple positioning with the augmentation. The increased cohesiveness of the gel and the texturization of the implant provides stability that tends to improve the expansion of the lower pole. These qualities allow the implant to "shape" the tight, constricted tissue rather than the tight tissue restricting and "shaping" the implant.

Additional Implant Characteristics

The ability to create different shapes to the breast has improved with the advancement in implant design. The performance of an implant is multifactorial and dependent on many features. The design of the implant, the shell, the gel cohesiveness, the gel-to-shell fill ratio, the gel cohesiveness, and the gel-to-shell interaction all affect the ultimate performance of the implant in vivo [14, 15]. Silicone implants are now available as fourth-generation and fifth-generation devices, based on the cohesiveness of the gel within the implant. All shaped devices are fifth-generation devices. Round implants can either be fourth generation, such as the Allergan Natrelle or Mentor MemoryGel implants, or fifth generation, such as the Sientra HSC and HSC+ or Allergan Soft touch and Cohesive implants. The greater the cohesiveness, the more stable the gel is within the device [15]. This can impact the appearance of the upper pole, stabilizing the sloping look of a shaped device or the rounded look of a round device. The fourth-generation gels will provide less stability in the implant shape, leading to a more natural upper pole or even failure to maintain the volume in the upper pole over time.

An additional feature has been to increase the gel-to-shell volume ratio, optimizing the fill of the implants. This can create a more stable volume in the upper pole as well, in addition to potentially reducing the amount of wrinkling seen with any given implant. All manufacturers have developed and offer implants with optimal fill ratios. In the augmentation mastopexy patients with more lax, thinner skin, the optimally filled implants have provided a much more predictable result with less upper pole failure and wrinkling of the implant.

Pocket Selection

Pocket selection for the augmentation mastopexy is often one of the most overlooked aspects and may have the greatest impact on the final results. The pocket choices include the submuscular, subfascial, and subglandular. The advantages and disadvantages of each are outlined in Table 2.4.

The dual-plane submuscular pocket is by far the most common implant pocket utilized (Fig. 2.9).

The dual-plane submuscular pocket is preferred if the upper pole pinch test is less than

Table 2.4 Advantages and disadvantages of pocket choices for the augmentation mastopexy

	Advantages	Disadvantages
Submuscular	• Lower capsular contracture rates • Enhance coverage of the implant • Reduced wrinkling visibility • Sloping natural upper pole • Enhanced support for the implant • Enhanced radiographic imaging with mammogram	• Animation deformity • Increased risk of implant superior malposition with waterfall deformity • Increased postoperative pain • Limited expansion of the lower pole of breast (required to expand constricted and ptotic breasts)
Subglandular	• Avoids implant deformation or distortion that can be seen in the subpectoral position • Enhances the improvement in the constricted or ptotic breast • Allows an easier dissection plane • Decreased postoperative discomfort • Allows access to the inframammary fold as the superficial and deep fascial components merge	• Less soft tissue coverage to disguise the implant • Increased visibility or palpability of implant with wrinkling or rippling • Higher capsular contracture rate • Less support and stabilization of the implants, especially shaped devices, compared to subfascial or submuscular pockets
Subfascial	• Avoids implant deformation or distortion (animation deformity) that can be seen in the subpectoral position • Provides additional soft tissue coverage between the implant and the skin as compared to the subglandular pocket • Provides additional support to minimize implant edge visibility and palpability seen most with subglandular placement • Fascia provides support of implant especially in the upper pole to minimize excess implant movement and potential rotation with shaped implants • Less postoperative pain as compared to submuscular placement • Provides a distinct layer separating the implant and overlying breast parenchyma	• Less soft tissue coverage compared to submuscular coverage • More challenging dissection to separate deep pectoral fascia from underlying muscle while keeping fascia intact • Higher rate of capsular contracture compared to submuscular

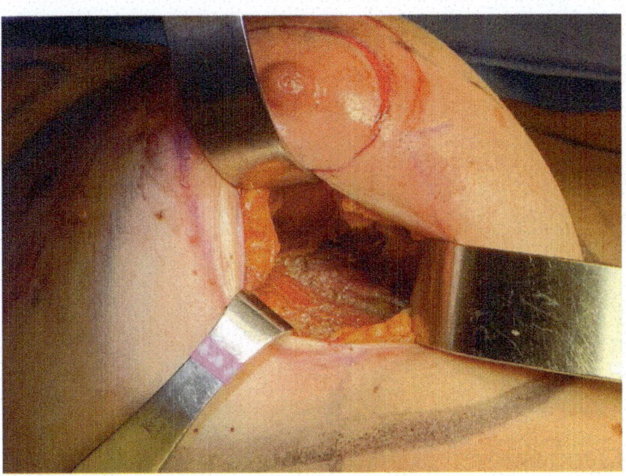

Fig. 2.9 Creation of the dual plane pocket by releasing the breast tissue from the underlying pectoralis major muscle

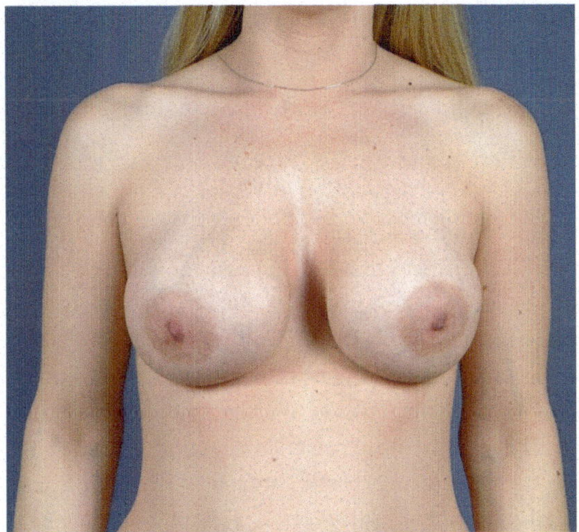

Fig. 2.10 Upper pole rippling due to minimal soft tissue coverage of the implant

2 cm in order to avoid upper pole implant visibility and wrinkling (Fig. 2.10).

The dual-plane pocket allows for submuscular pocket with additional coverage and support in the upper portion of the breast while being subglandular and allowing for greater expansion in the lower poles of the breast (Fig. 2.11) [25]. Interestingly, the tighter or looser the lower pole, the greater the level of dual plane needed. The constricted, lower pole breast requires greater dual plane, level 2 or 3, to allow for maximal expansion of the tight lower pole.

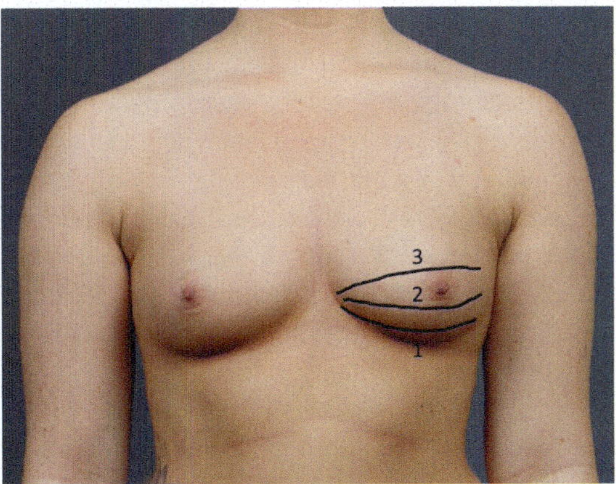

Fig. 2.11 Dual plane levels. Dual plane 1 is complete division the pectoralis major muscle (PMM) along the IMF. Dual plane 2 is release of the breast tissue off the PMM up to the lower areola. Dual plane 3 is release of the breast tissue off of the PMM up to the upper border of the areola

Muscle in the lower pole would limit the amount of expansion possible in this tight tissue envelope. The additional parenchymal exposure with the dual planes allows for parenchymal expansion techniques such as radial scoring. The very lax, loose breast also requires greater expansion for correction. Whereas one might think this is not necessarily due to the overlying mastopexy that is capable of tightening the tissue over the implant, the very lax breast even after a mastopexy will often fall off of the under expanded lower pole and implant, leading to a waterfall deformity. The ability of the implant to have some influence over the overlying breast tissue is an important and yet often misunderstood concepts for achieving long-term success in augmentation mastopexy. The most lax and thin breast envelopes, such as the weight loss patients, require the lifting effect of the implant even in the face of a mastopexy to avoid a waterfall deformity with time.

A subfascial pocket is possible if the upper pole pinch is 2 cm or greater. In the author's opinion, the subglandular pocket should be reserved for those with upper pole pinch of 3 cm or greater. These are only suggested guidelines and many other factors contribute to pocket decisions, including not only the thickness of the soft tissue coverage but also the quality of the tissue. Additionally, the implant decision impacts the appropriateness of placing the implant above the muscle. There is good evidence that when a subglandular/subfascial pocket is utilized, a textured device has a lower capsular contracture rate compared to a smooth implant. Likewise, the size of the implant can impact the development of a stretch deformity when placed without muscular support. Finally, implants placed above the muscle have less coverage in the upper pole compared to submuscular implants. Thus, when above the muscle, implants with greater cohesiveness, optimal fills, and possible texture provide a more optimal implant for limiting lower pole stretch over time and maintaining upper pole volume.

Mastopexy Technique

When determined that a one-stage augmentation mastopexy is deemed appropriate, the approach to the mastopexy is based on the preoperative evaluation. The assessment of the level of ptosis (see Table 2.1) guides the surgeon in assessing the need for NAC elevation, as well as skin envelope reduction and possibly parenchymal excision.

Circumareolar

Although performed less often, patients with borderline ptosis, grade 1 ptosis or pseudoptosis (N-IMF under maximal stretch 10 cm), low NAC (such as constricted breast deformity), or tuberous breast deformity may benefit from a circumareolar mastopexy. This can elevate the NAC modestly (2 cm or less) and can reduce the areolar diameter. There should be minimal overhang of breast over the fold and limited horizontal laxity. The circumareolar mastopexy should be used very selectively, as it can create widening and flattening of the breast, which may prove beneficial in a tuberous breast deformity but undesirable in a deflated, flattened breast. This approach is mostly correcting the NAC and improve the shape of the NAC and breast but with little ability to actually "lift" the breast.

Circumvertical

Patients with moderate ptosis, grade 1 or 2, requiring NAC elevation of usually less than 4 cm, with modest amounts of breast overhanging the fold can be addressed with a circumvertical mastopexy with or without removal of a small amount of skin along the fold (horizontal wedge). These patients tend to have more horizontal laxity requiring breast narrowing with only a modest amount of reduction in the vertical component.

Circumvertical with Inverted-T Skin Excision

For patients with more severe ptosis, grade 2 or 3, with significant vertical excess and overhang over the fold, a circumvertical with inverted-T skin excision is more appropriate to achieve optimal results. The greater the vertical excess and laxity, the greater the horizontal wedge and the longer the incision becomes along the inframammary fold.

When planning the type of mastopexy, it is important to distinguish between the pedicle design and the skin excision design of the mastopexy [11]. In augmentation mastopexy, the design of the more ptotic breast is always a circumvertical approach with the superior or occasional the superomedial pedicle as the pedicle blood supply. The only difference in the approach is whether skin needs to be excised along the fold. Thus, even in the more ptotic breasts with significant laxity requiring an inverted-T skin pattern excision, the parenchymal and pedicle design is still a circumvertical approach with a superior pedicle. In these patients, if the breasts are heavy with excessive ptotic parenchyma, a lower pole parenchymal resection along with the skin excision is optimal to reduce the likelihood of recurrent ptosis postoperatively [26].

Lower Pole Mastopexy

There is an occasional patient, especially in secondary cases, in which the NAC is in satisfactory position but a significant amount of glandular ptosis or pseudoptosis is present. These patients may benefit from simply an inframammary fold resection (smile mastopexy) or vertical-horizontal resection (sailboat mastopexy) without transposing the NAC [27]. This can address both vertical and horizontal laxity without jeopardizing NAC circulation and placing an unnecessary scar around the areola.

Operative Technique

Preoperative Markings

Appropriate preoperative markings provide a roadmap and are essential to planning and performing an augmentation mastopexy (Fig. 2.12). The markings guide the surgeon in providing symmetrical NAC placement and mastopexy design. The patient is sitting upright during the markings. A line is initially drawn along the midline of the breasts and bilaterally down the meridians. The meridian lines bisect the breast equally and may not intersect through the nipple if there is NAC malposition. The inframammary folds are then drawn, noting any asymmetries to be addressed at surgery. The position of the IMF is then drawn on the anterior breast through the meridian incision. This augmentation mastopexy is based on a superior pedicle blood supply and is not dependent on the final skin excision pattern.

Decision on nipple placement is performed is based on the location of the fold and expectation on the location of the new lifted breasts with an underlying implant. This can be approximated by simulating the mastopexy and identifying the probable location of the NAC. The nipple position is marked along the breast meridian at or within 2–4 cm of the reflected inframammary fold (Fig. 2.13).

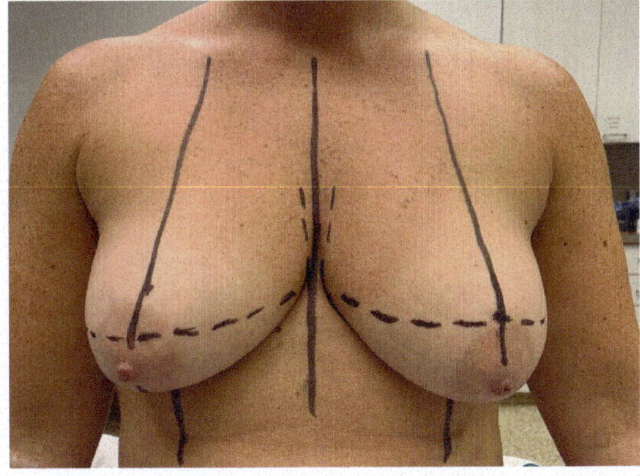

Fig. 2.12 Preoperative markings showing the midline of the chest, the breast meridian, the IMF, and the transposed/reflected inframammary fold (dotted line)

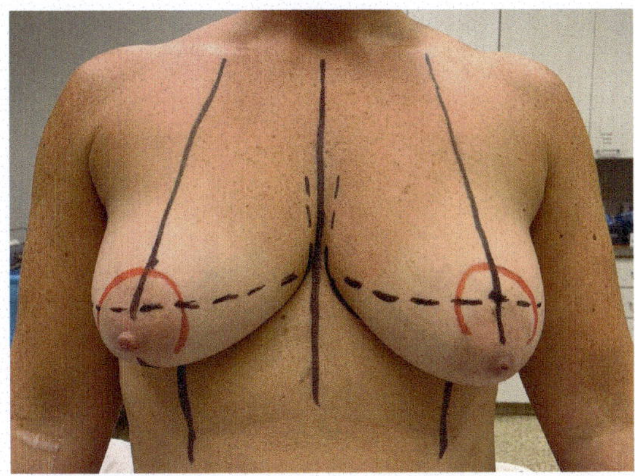

Fig. 2.13 The new NAC position marked within 2–4 cm of the reflected IMF on the breast meridian

In the circumareolar approach, the proposed location of the new areolar opening is marked, starting approximately 2 cm above the nipple position and 6–8 cm above the inframammary fold based on implant size. An oval line is then drawn from the two points extending around the areola to create the desired shape and skin excision.

Vertical Mastopexy Technique

When a vertical or inverted-T mastopexy is planned, the areola is drawn from the planned superior areola opening extending around the areola to produce an areolar opening of approximately 42 millimeters. The breasts are then rotated medially and laterally to mark the location of the vertical incisions, recognizing that the placement of the implant will add volume, thus requiring less skin excision than would be required with mastopexy designed without an implant (Fig. 2.14).

If the vertical limbs are deemed excessively long, the design can be modified to include additional skin excision around the areola (circum-

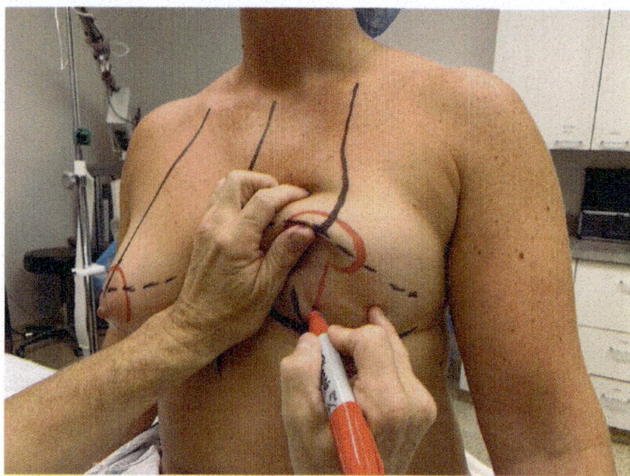

Fig. 2.14 Left breast rotated medially to mark location of lateral vertical incision shown in red

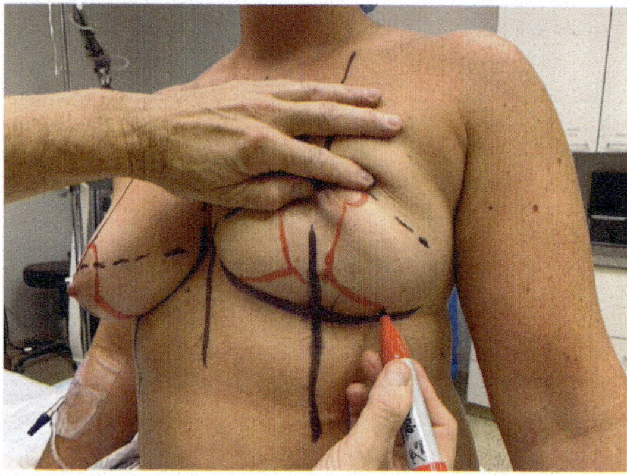

Fig. 2.15 Preoperative drawing of anticipated horizontal wedge excision shown as red line above the IMF to shorten the vertical limb of the mastopexy

vertical mastopexy) or along the inframammary fold (circumvertical with horizontal wedge excision) (Fig. 2.15).

Patients with greater ptosis will often require more significant excision of skin and elevation of the NAC. This can range from a long wise-pattern excision down to a very short horizontal wedge based on the amount of skin excess. These markings are made along the inframammary fold and intersect with a line drawn from the vertical limbs extending in a curved fashion down to the fold markings. When planning an augmentation mastopexy, these drawings should be conservative allowing for adjustments once the implant has been placed. All the markings made preoperatively are made as a guideline for the operation, but the final NAC placement and skin excision required will be determined in surgery after the breast implant has been placed.

Surgical Technique

The patient is placed on the operating room table with the arms secured to the sides at 45–60° (Fig. 2.16).

Once the patient is prepped with Chloraprep and draped appropriately, the markings and incision location are confirmed and reinforced with a surgical pen to avoid loss of markings during the prep. The operative field is then injected with 50 cc per side of local anesthetic of 0.25% lidocaine, 0.125% Marcaine, 1:400,000 epinephrine (Table 2.5, Fig. 2.17).

Each breast is placed under maximal stretch, and the areolas are marked with a 42-mm cookie-cutter (range 38–45 mm depending on desired aesthetics) and incised with a 15-blade scalpel (Fig. 2.18).

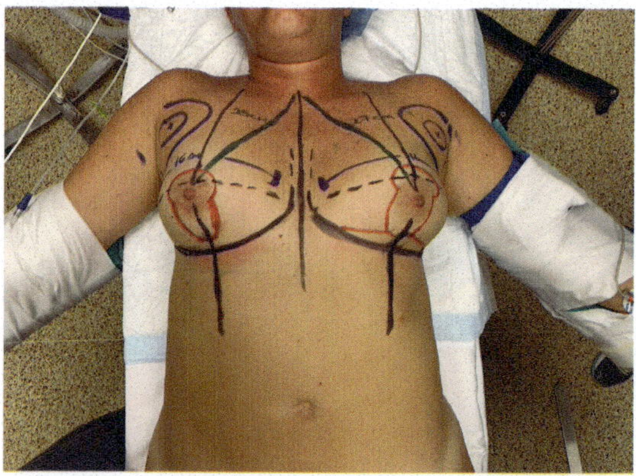

Fig. 2.16 Patient positioning on the table with the arms secured and at the side approximately 45–60°

Table 2.5 Concentration of breast local anesthetic

Breast local anesthetic formula	
½% Lidocaine plain	25 ml
½% Lidocaine/1:200,000 epinephrine	25 ml
½% Bupivicaine/1:200,000 epinephrine	25 ml
Injectable saline	25 ml
Total concentration	*Total volume*
¼% Lidocaine, 1/8% bupivicaine, 1:400,000 epinephrine	100 ml

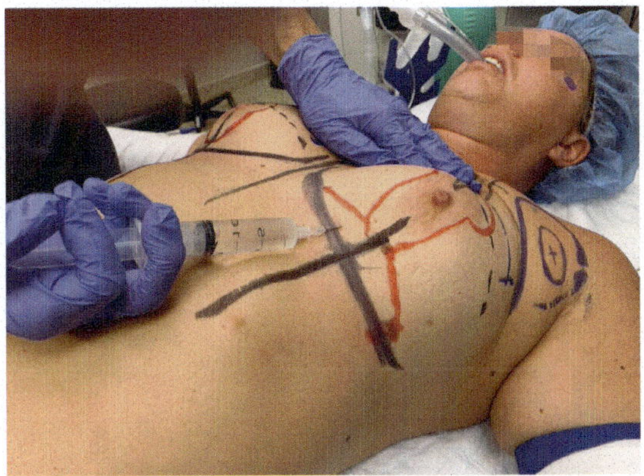

Fig. 2.17 Injection of breast local analgesic using a 20-cc syringe and a spinal needle

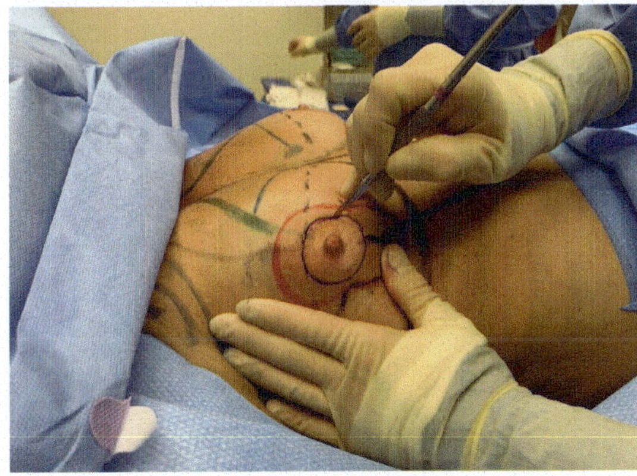

Fig. 2.18 Incision of the NAC with 15-blade scalpel

Pocket Development

Once the areolas are incised, access to the breast pocket is determined. For circumareolar mastopexies, the access is either through the inferior areola in the area of planned de-epithelization or through a counter-incision in the IMF. The advantages of going through the areola is eliminating the need for an additional scar in the IMF. It also has been proposed that when lowering the fold, the dissection from above can allow for fold lowering incrementally, obviating the need to determine its new position preoperatively. However, the preferred access currently is with an IMF incision. This provides improved exposure and visualization of the pocket, is associated with lower capsular contracture rates, and allows for IMF control sutures to be placed to stabilize the new fold position. In the circumareolar approach, the skin edges are retracted inferiorly and superiorly and dissection is carried down toward the pectoralis fascia either directly through the breast tissue (transparenchymal) or inferiorly under the skin (subcutaneous) until the fascia is reached at the fold (Fig. 2.19).

The author prefers the transparenchymal approach. If access is through an IMF counter incision, the dissection is carried through Scarpa's fascia leaving a small cuff on the inferior incision, and then dissected under the breast directly onto the pectoralis fascia (Fig. 2.20).

When a vertical or inverted-T skin incision is planned, access to the breast pocket can be made via the periareolar, vertical, or the inframammary approach. However, a vertical access approach is utilized in the vast majority of cases. The breast is divided down the midline extending from the inferior areola to at least 2 cm above the inframammary fold to gain access to the desired pocket (Fig. 2.21).

It is extremely important to not carry this incision all the way down to the fold because this lower area of the breast, the "No-Go Zone," will provide a protective cuff of tissue during closure (Fig. 2.22).

Once through the breast tissue, the pocket is created based on preoperative decision-making.

Submuscular Dual-Plane Pocket

Dissection is carried down toward the chest wall while maintaining a constant upward retraction of the breast tissue, ultimately exposing the lateral edge of the pectoralis muscle. The upward retraction of the breast tissue is key as the suspensory ligaments of the breast will concomi-

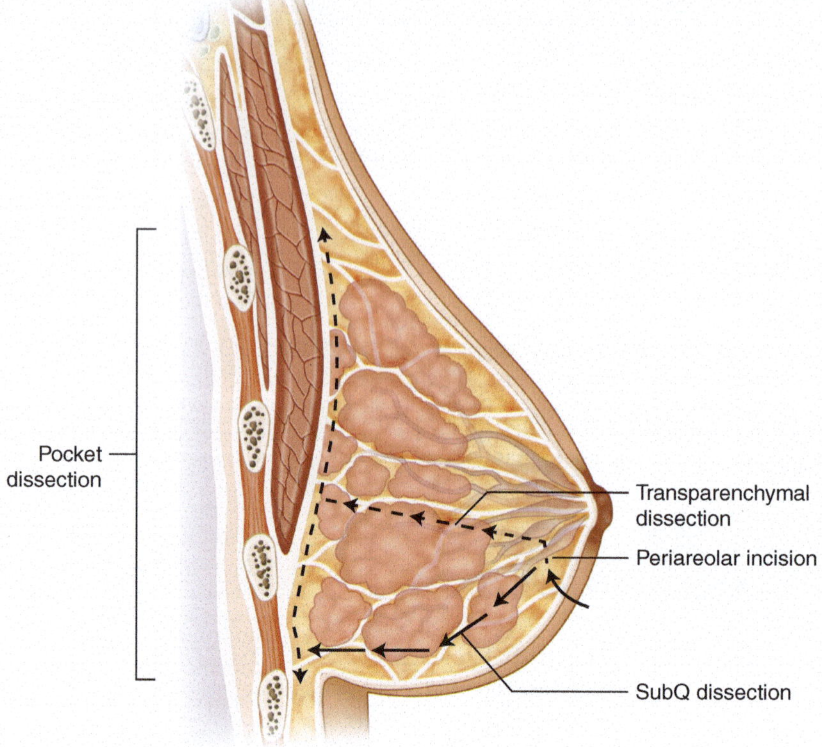

Fig. 2.19 Illustration of the periareolar incision with dissection in either the subcutaneous or transparenchymal plane

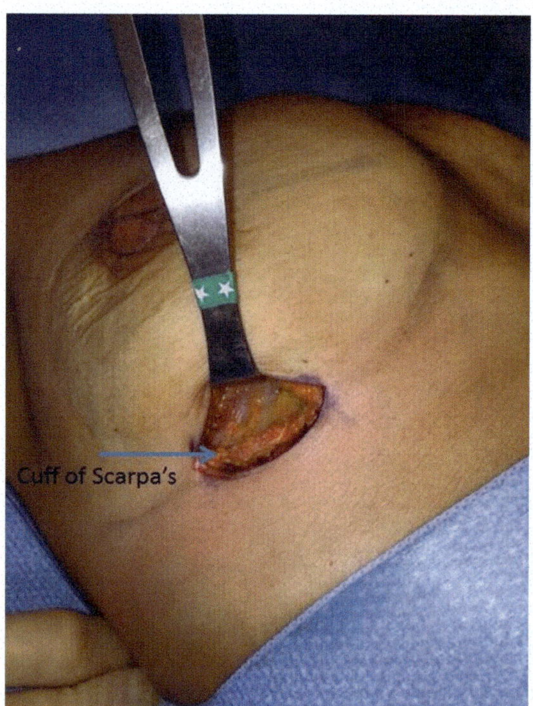

Fig. 2.20 Small cuff of Scarpa's fascia at the IMF incision

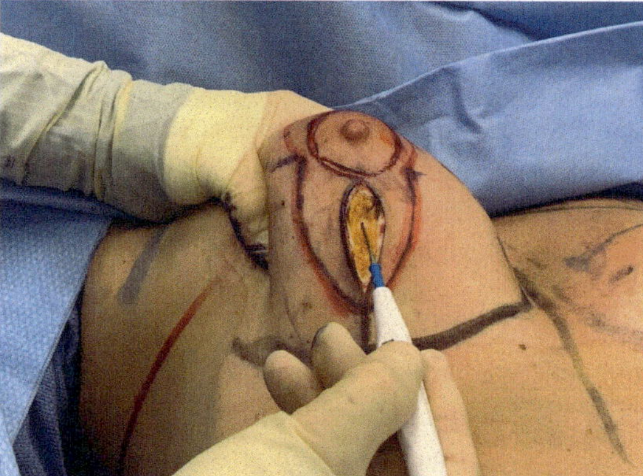

Fig. 2.21 Vertical access approach to the breast, incision is made inferior to the NAC

tantly elevate the muscle. It is imperative to not cut the muscle unless you can elevate the muscle off the chest wall. Inability to elevate the muscle most likely indicates that the identified muscle is actually not the pectoralis, but rather the serratus, rectus, or an intercostal muscle. Once the lateral border of the pectoralis is identified, the

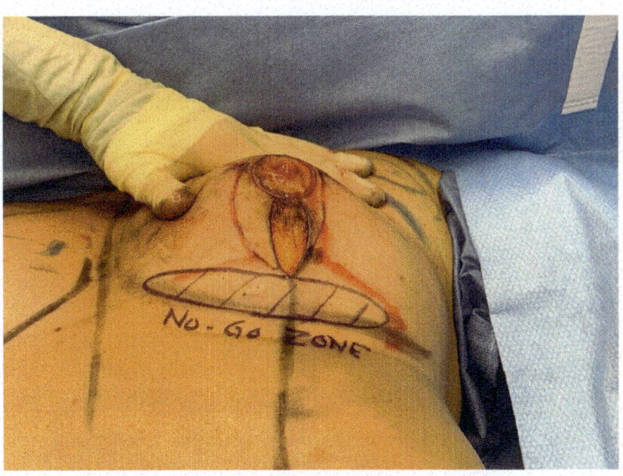

Fig. 2.22 Vertical dissection to just above the IMF leaving a cuff of tissue (no-go zone) to protect implant at the T-point

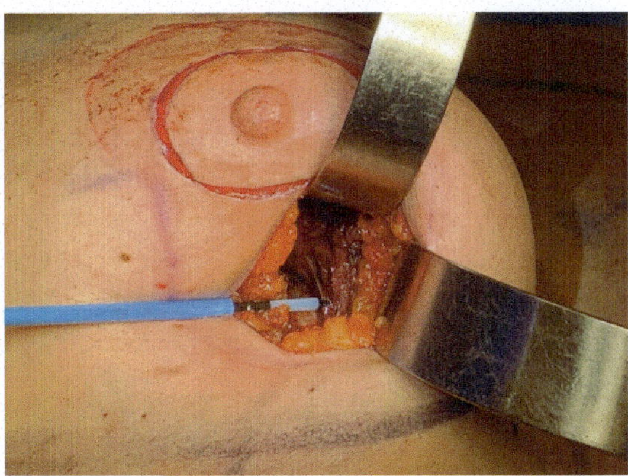

Fig. 2.23 Dissection of pectoralis major staying at least 1 cm above the IMF

fascia is incised to expose the underlying muscle. After the subpectoral space is entered, dissection is carried upward centrally to the superior extent of the pocket. Dissection is then carried laterally just superficial to the pectoralis minor and serratus anterior until the lateral border of the pocket is reached. Lateral pocket dissection should be performed bluntly with minimal cautery to avoid injury to the lateral cutaneous nerves resulting in sensory changes to the NAC. Especially important in augmentation mastopexy cases, dissection of the pocket laterally should be minimized to facilitate optimal medial projection of the implant.

The pectoralis is then released along the planned IMF, staying 1 cm superior to the fold to account for caudal muscle descent (Fig. 2.23).

Dissection directly at the fold will often lead to a fold that is lower than planned as the muscle retracts inferiorly. As you carry your dissection medially along the IMF, it is critically important to stop the dissection at the most medial extent along the sternum. Preservation of the most caudal attachment of the pectoralis muscle at the *transition point* (TP) along the sternum is critical to minimize the chance of window shading of the pectoralis with subsequent medial implant exposure and animation deformities. A *transition zone* (TZ) of tapered muscle release connects the transition point to the main body of medial pectoral muscle along the sternum (Fig. 2.24).

The extent of the pocket is completed by defining the medial pectoral border and dividing all of the accessory slips of pectoralis muscle that insert along the ribs, preserving only the main body of the muscle as it inserts along the sternum. Dividing these muscles slips with electrocautery instead of blunt dissection improves postoperative cleavage, weakens the pectoralis muscle action on the implant, and maintains hemostasis. This division of the inferior pectoralis muscle just above the IMF during initial pocket dissection creates a level-1 dual plane. Thus, all submuscular pockets where the muscle is released inferiorly are actually dual-plane pockets, as the segment between the caudal edge of the divided muscle and the inframammary fold is subglandular.

The level of dual plane required varies, and each surgery can be tailored to provide the optimal level based on soft-tissue requirements and implant selection (Table 2.6). The greater the amount of breast parenchyma or breast laxity, the greater the level of dual plane. It is this creation of a lower pole subglandular pocket that allows for an optimal breast–implant interface and soft tissue re-draping. In augmentation mastopexy, the breast–implant relationship is improved with the overlying mastopexy. However, even with a mastopexy, failure to optimize the breast–implant interface during surgery can lead to a waterfall deformity with the breast sliding off the implant.

If IMF lowering is required, it can be more challenging in the submuscular pocket as it is

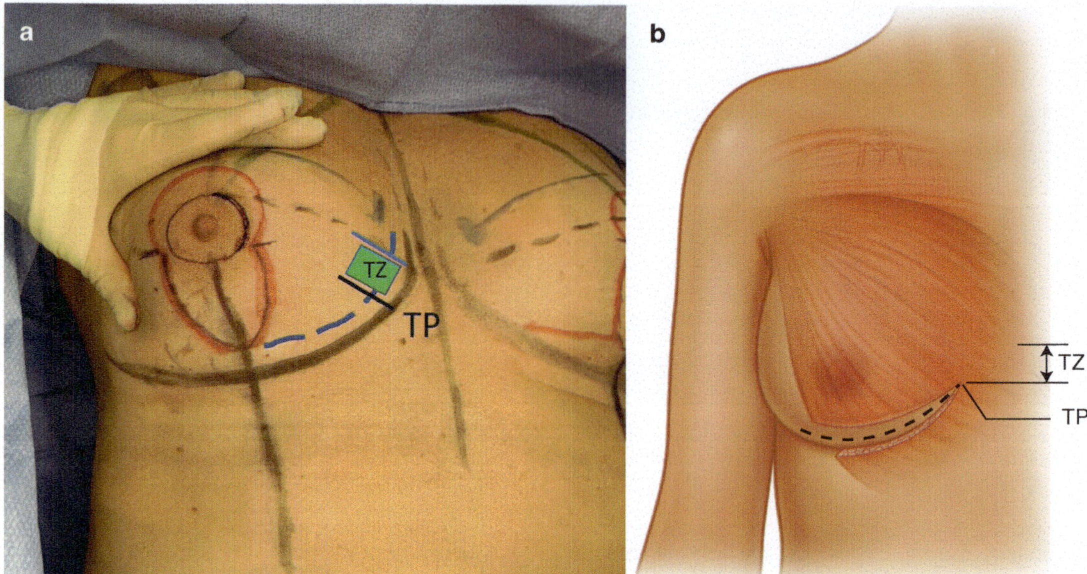

Fig. 2.24 (a) TP is the transition point where the pectoralis major is no longer completely released from costal attachments (dark black vertical line). The dotted blue line represents pectoralis muscle release 1 cm above the IMF. The TZ (green shaded region) is the transition zone as the pectoralis major is thinned from the TP to the sternum. (b) Schematic showing the TP (transition point) and TZ (transition zone)

Table 2.6 Dual-plane types

Dual-plane type	Description
Type I	Complete division of the pectoralis major along the IMF
Type II	Same as I plus pectoralis is released from overlying gland and allowed to slide to about the lower border of the areola
Type III	Same as type I plus greater release of the pectoralis from the gland, allowing it to slide to about the upper border of the areola

tempting to carry the dissection under the muscle along the chest wall to lower the fold. The dissection along the chest wall at the level of the fold is deep to the suspensory ligament structures that create the IMF. IMF lowering in the subpectoral pocket requires transitioning into a more superficial subglandular plane above the pectoralis fascia to lower the IMF. Dissection deep to the pectoral fascia will likely result in a lowered fold with persistence of the native fold structure, resulting in a double-bubble deformity (Fig. 2.25).

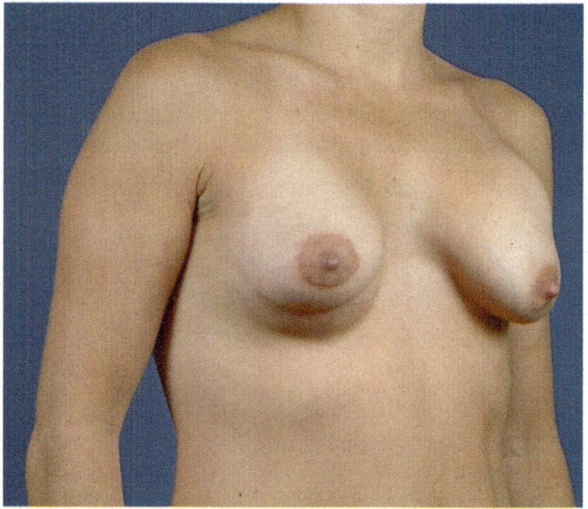

Fig. 2.25 Oblique view showing the double-bubble deformity of the right breast and a waterfall deformity of the left breast

This is more likely when dissection begins from above, such as a periareolar or transaxillary approach. Fortunately, when using an IMF incision, the dissection below the native fold begins in the subcutaneous plane until the pectoralis muscle is reached, resulting in appropriate obliteration of the native fold at the correct level.

Subfascial Pocket (Fig. 2.26)
As you dissect toward the chest wall maintaining a constant upward retraction of the breast tissue, the pectoralis major will be exposed with its overlying fascia. Elevation beneath the deep pectoral fascia and overlying breast tissue exposes the pectoral muscle fibers devoid of fascia. The elevation of the pectoralis fascia can start at the IMF and move superiorly or can be elevated with the breast tissue centrally and then dissected superiorly and inferiorly in development of the pocket. Importantly, the inframammary fold is a fusion of the deep fascia attached to the pectoralis and the superficial fascia of the breast. Take care to prevent disruption of the inframammary fold as the inferior edge of the fascia elevated. The inferior extent of the pectoralis fascia is thin, and elevation is best carried out with the cut current of the electrocautery. Continued upward retraction of the breast will elevate the fascial plane. The fascia is left attached to the underlying breast tissue and elevated as a single unit. The dissection is carried superiorly, medial and lateral to create the desired pocket. As with any breast augmentation, pocket control is key. Avoid over-dissection of your pocket laterally to optimize medial projection of the implant and minimize lateralization of the implant. Subfascial implants have less lateral drift compared to submuscular implants because they lack the lateral action of the forceful pectoralis muscle contraction. As the dissection is carried medially, be aware of the midline to avoid pocket over-dissection which could lead to symmastia. The fascia is adherent to the underlying pectoralis muscle as the sternum is approached and will provide some limitation to medial over dissection compared to the subglandular pocket. Importantly, if IMF lowering is needed, the dissection is transitioned into the subglandular pocket as the attachments creating the fold are superficial to the deep pectoral fascia.

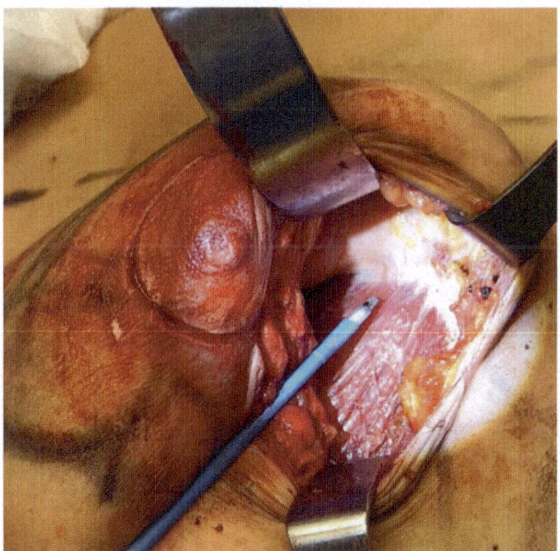

Fig. 2.26 Subfascial pocket creation by elevating the pectoralis major fascia off the underlying muscle. In this image, the overlying breast tissue is still adherent to the fascia

Subglandular Pocket (Fig. 2.27)
The elevation of the subglandular pocket is superficial to the pectoralis fascia. As you dissect toward the chest wall, a continued upward retraction of the breast will elevate the breast and its thin underlying fascia as a single unit leaving the pectoralis fascia attached to the muscle. The fascia is visualized over the pectoralis muscle as a dull covering obscuring the appearance of the fleshy muscle fibers. The dissection is carried superiorly, medial and lateral to create the desired pocket. The inframammary fold is

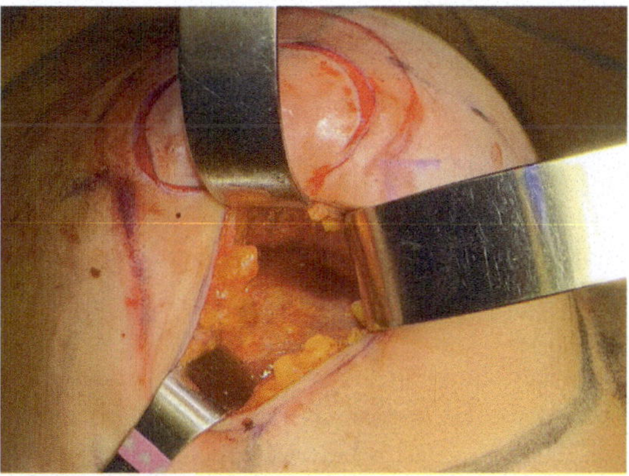

Fig. 2.27 Subglandular pocket creation by elevating the breast tissue off the pectoralis major muscle. The "shiny" pectoralis major deep fascia is still adherent to the underlying muscle as the breast tissue is being elevated

a fusion of the deep fascia attached to the pectoralis and the superficial fascia of the breast. Take care to prevent disruption of the inframammary fold as the breast is elevated off of the pectoralis fascia. Avoid over-dissection of your pocket laterally to optimize medial projection of the implant and minimize lateralization of the implant. Subglandular implants have less lateral drift compared to submuscular implants because they lack the lateral action of the forceful pectoralis muscle contraction. As you carry your dissection medially in the subglandular plane, the midline can quickly be violated due to the lack of sternal muscle attachment that limits dissection in the submuscular plan. Over-dissection can lead to medial migration of the implant and the potential for postoperative symmastia. This is especially true when the chest wall is concave or slanting medially, and special caution with limited medial dissection is warranted in these cases. If IMF lowering is indicated, the dissection is more easily accomplished as the subglandular plane dissection inferiorly is in the appropriate plane to lower and obliterate the native fold.

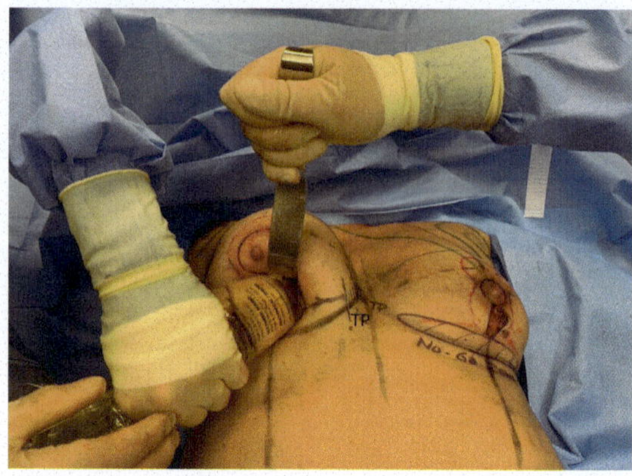

Fig. 2.28 Use of the Keller funnel to insert the implant into the breast pocket

Implant Placement

Once the pocket is developed, hemostasis is established. Prospective hemostasis with control of any blood staining during the dissection is optimal. The pocket is irrigated with the triple antibiotic solution/betadine solution (1 g of cefazolin sodium, 80 mg gentamycin, 50 cc betadine mixed in 500 mL of normal saline) and a final hemostasis check is done. The implants are soaked in the irrigation solution before insertion. Gloves are changed and rinsed with the irrigation solution to remove any residue. The implant is then placed into the pocket with the assistance of an insertion sleeve such as the Keller funnel (Fig. 2.28). The use of the insertion sleeve is even more beneficial in an augmentation mastopexy surgery as the implant is passed through either the circumareolar or vertical incision in the vast majority of patients.

These access incisions require the implant to pass through the bacteria-laden breast tissue. The insertion sleeve provides a "minimal-touch" technique that is associated with lower capsular contracture rates [28, 29].

The insertion sleeve is placed deep into the pocket to allow passage with minimal to no contact with the surrounding breast tissue. The opening of the funnel should be cut large enough to allow easy egress of the implant through the funnel. This is easily confirmed by passing the implant with irrigation solution through the funnel prior to insertion. The implant orientation is then confirmed in the funnel, and a maneuver of squeezing the implant through the funnel with pressure exerted on the back of the funnel allows the implant to slip into the breast pocket.

Once the implant is in the pocket, a finger-assisted assessment and manipulation of the implant within the pocket is necessary to confirm its proper placement and assure appropriate re-draping of the breast parenchyma over the implant. This maneuver is especially important with textured devices, either round or shaped, as these implants are less mobile and less likely to stretch the pocket and, thus, a distortion or wrinkling of the implant in a tight pocket may be permanent if not resolved before closure.

When using a shaped device, it is imperative to assure appropriate placement of the implant and to confirm the orientation marks or tabs are correctly positioned (Fig. 2.29).

Repeated removal and insertions of the implant should be avoided to minimize implant or incision damage, potential contamination, and

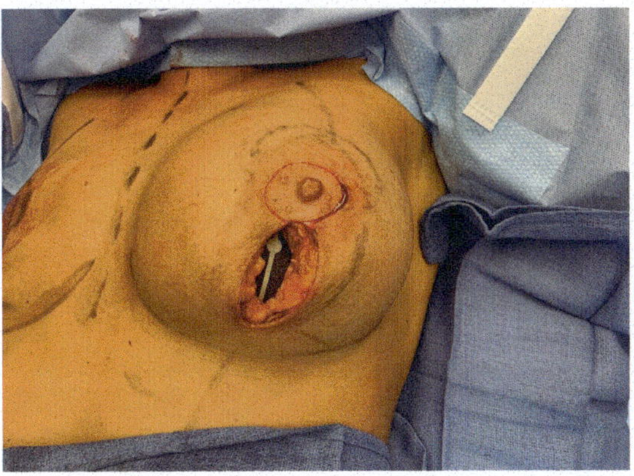

Fig. 2.29 White stripe to maintain the vertical orientation of the shaped implant

pocket over dissection. This is especially important with shaped implants, as a stretched pocket from over manipulation could lead to implant rotation postoperatively.

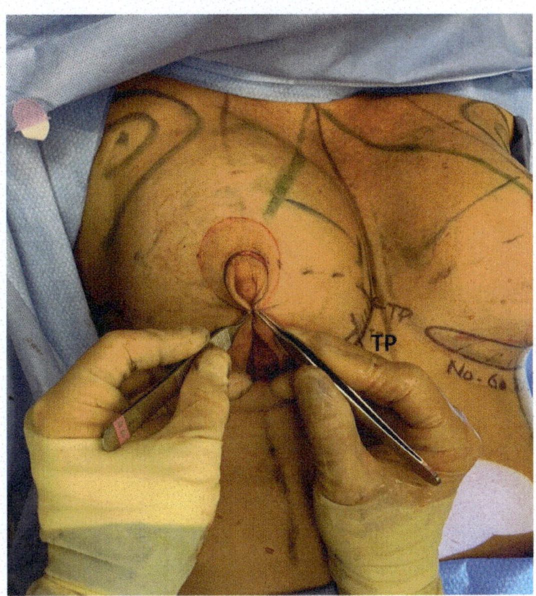

Fig. 2.30 Tailor tacking of the breast with staples. The medial and lateral vertical limbs are brought together and stapled in a descending fashion beginning at the 6 o'clock position of the NAC

Tailor-Tacking (Figs. 2.30, 2.31, and 2.32)

Once the implant is in the pocket and oriented appropriately, the final planning of the mastopexy is carried out. Tailor-tacking is a critical step in designing the optimal breast shape. With the circumareolar approach, the areola is stapled to the outer circle and adjusted to create the desired shape prior to de-epithelialization. In the vertical or inverted-T approach, starting usually at what will be the new inferior areola location (6 o'clock position), the medial and lateral vertical limbs are brought together and stapled in a descending fashion, adjusting by tightening a little more or a little less to create the desired lower pole breast shape. If a vertical approach only, the planned excision tapers down to the fold. The length of the lower pole skin (distance from the inferior areola to IMF) varies based on the size of implant and amount of breast parenchyma that is present. For most augmentation mastopexies, this length is generally 6–8 cm. If this distance is excessive when tailor-tacking, two options exist: expand the circumareolar opening to encompass more of the vertical length (circumvertical approach)

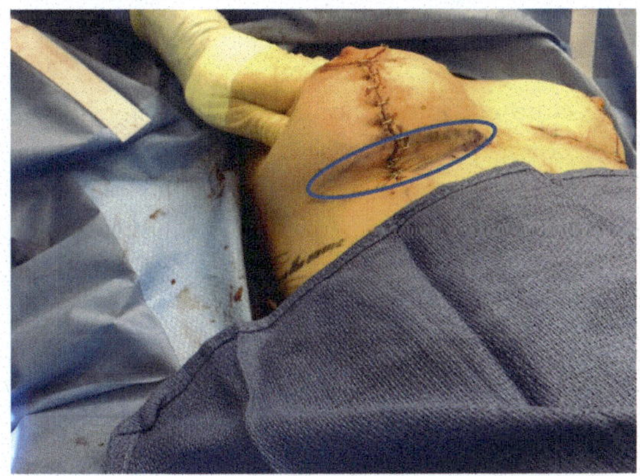

Fig. 2.31 Blue circle estimates the resection size of the horizontal wedge of tissue to deal with the vertical excess present at the time of tailor-tacking

or remove a horizontal wedge of skin at the fold to shorten the vertical limb. This often is a small wedge of skin leaving a short horizontal scar (has been referred to as owl's feet) or extended laterally as J-type mastopexy. If the vertical excess is significant, the horizontal wedge excision will create an inverted-T pattern. With the patient in the upright position and the arms extended at 45°, breast shape and symmetry are confirmed.

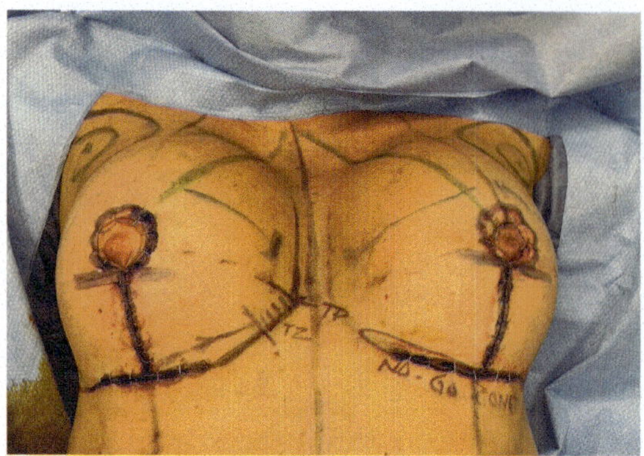

Fig. 2.32 Both breasts are tailor-tacked with staples, including the horizontal wedge resections

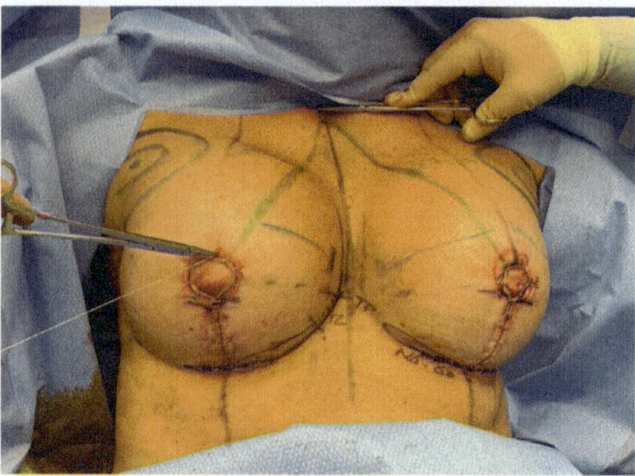

Fig. 2.33 Confirming the NAC placement is symmetrical using the top-down approach from sternal notch to the top of the areola

Adjustments are made if necessary, until the results are optimal.

Important to mention, once the tacking is complete, a final decision on placement of the NAC must be made. There is flexibility as no skin has been excised at this time. The areolar can be positioned higher or lower to optimize breast shape, placing the NAC centrally along the median of the breast at the point of maximal projection. When considering NAC placement, confirmation can be performed from bottom up, top down, or both. "Top down" refers to the distance from the sternal notch to the top of the areola (or nipple) and "bottom up" refers to the distance from the IMF to the inferior areola (or nipple). During tailor-tacking, it is helpful to confirm NAC position and symmetry using both techniques (Figs. 2.33 and 2.34).

Once confirmed, the patient is placed supine, and the tailor-tacking is marked with methylene blue or permanent marker identifying the planned incision lines.

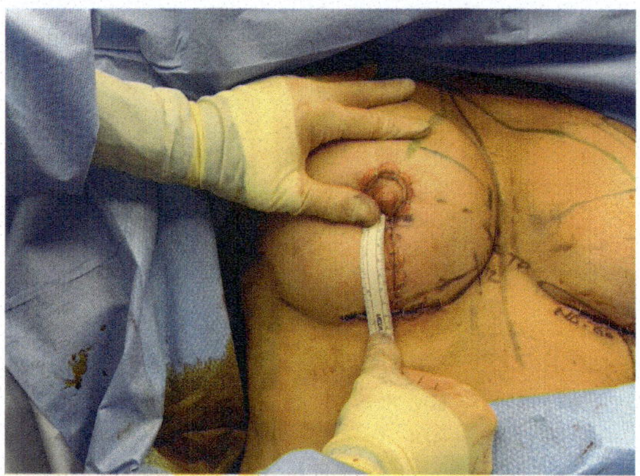

Fig. 2.34 Bottom-up measurement of the NAC, which is between 6 and 8 cm from the IMF to the inferior border of the NAC

Breast Flap and Pedicle Dissection

In the circumareolar approach, the area between the areola and outer circle is de-epithelialized. Although an IMF counter-incision is the preferred access for the augmentation, if the periareolar access was used, then the deep breast tissue must first be closed with an absorbable 2-0 Vicryl. The dermis is then cauterized for maximal shrinkage (Fig. 2.35).

The dermis is either left intact or incised just at the periphery to create a small ledge to facilitate closure. A purse string suture of 3-0 Gortex is placed in a wagon wheel pattern (Fig. 2.36).

In the vertical augmentation mastopexy technique, the superior pedicle is preferred. The incisions are outlined with a scalpel, insuring not to cut deeply into the dermis. The periareolar region is de-epithelialized (Fig. 2.37). The incisions are then made full thickness through the dermis along all of the scored skin. However, in the superior areola, the dermis is left intact (from 8 o'clock to 4 o'clock) as the superior dermal pedicle.

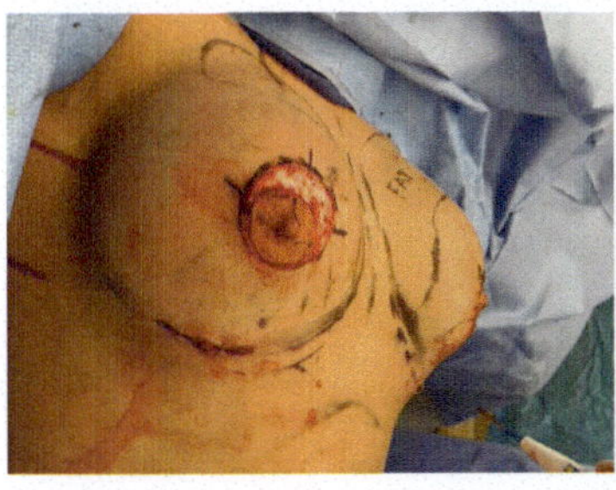
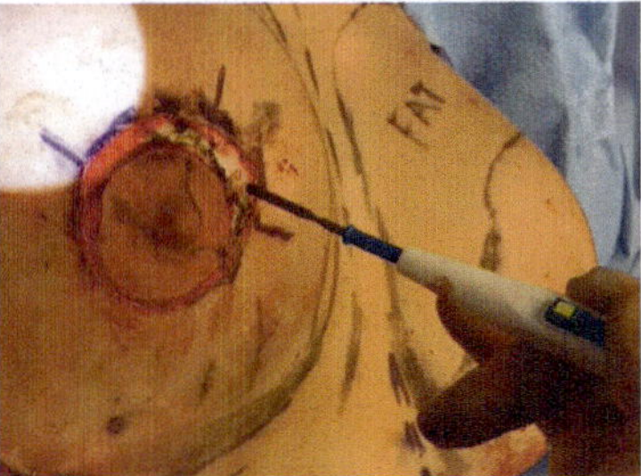

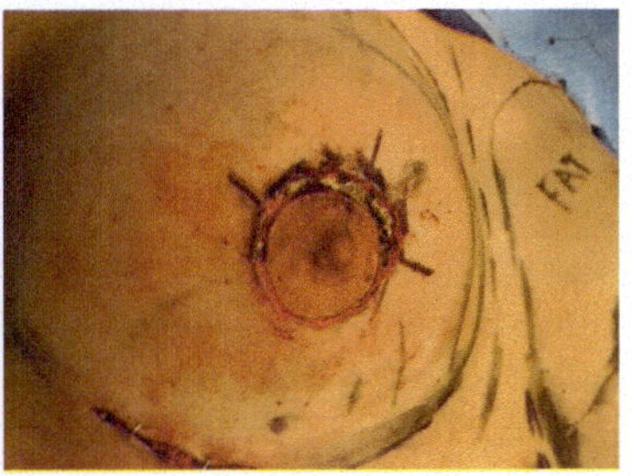

Fig. 2.35 Dermis is cauterized to shrink the periareolar tissue and facilitate a tension free closure

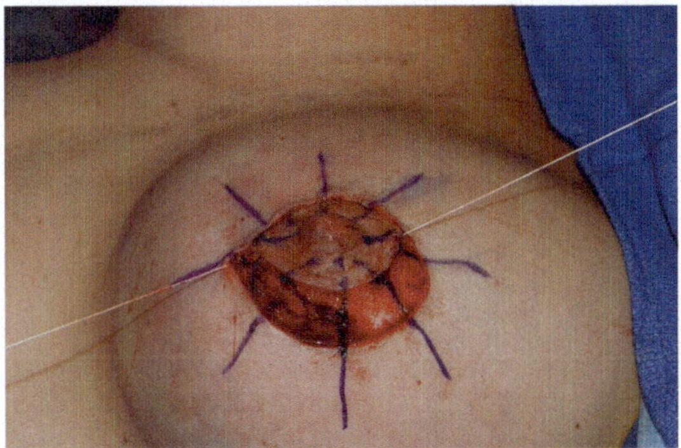

Fig. 2.36 Wagon wheel closure of the NAC with a 3-0 Gortex

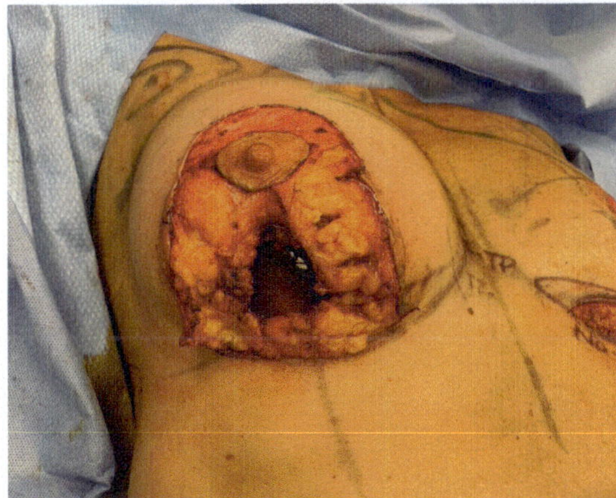

Fig. 2.37 Periareolar and vertical limb are de-epithelialized. Note that the dermis around the NAC is left intact from 8 to 4 o'clock to maintain NAC perfusion

Lower Pole De-bulking

If the patient is extremely thin, such as in a revision surgery or a patient with paper-thin skin, the vertical skin ± the horizontal skin is de-epithelialized and maintained for additional coverage and support with the mastopexy. However, most patients with ptotic breasts have significant amounts of excess skin and breast tissue in the lower pole. In these patients, de-bulking of the lower pole is probably the single most important step in the procedure to reduce likelihood of recurrent ptosis. Breast flaps along the medial and lateral vertical incisions are initially created, staying approximately 2 cm or greater in thickness. Located centrally is the lower pole segment of breast tissue located from the areola to the IMF within the vertical incisions. This tissue is aggressively de-bulked to reduce lower pole stretch over time with recurrent ptosis. It also reduces the tension on the lower pole mastopexy flap closure. When de-bulking the lower pole, the anterior tissue is removed preserving a posterior lamellae of breast tissue and posterior breast fascia. It is especially important to maintain the "no-go zone" cuff of breast tissue located above the IMF as this creates the floor for the implant and provides protection for the implant if skin breakdown occurs at the level of the IMF (Fig. 2.38).

Deep Fascial Sling

Once the pedicle has been developed and appropriate skin and breast tissue removed, closure of the breast pocket is performed. However, this step is extremely important to creating a lamellar closure over the implant and developing the shape of the lower pole. As in all mastopexy techniques, controlling the lower pole of the breast through parenchymal shaping and not skin tightening provides increased stability of the results over time. Starting inferiorly, which is just above the "no-go" cuff of breast tissue, the lateral and medial pillars are brought together at the most posterior aspect of the breast just superficial to the implant with a running 2-0 Vicryl suture. This 2-0 Vicryl running suture carries the closure superiorly toward the NAC, continually tightening the lateral pillar and the medial pillar to create the desired lower pole shape. Therefore, this step is not just closing over the implant, it is parenchymal shaping in a vertical fashion to control overall breast shape and vertical projection. This closure additionally adds an additional layer of closure, protecting the underlying implant (Fig. 2.39).

Once the breast pocket is closed, any additional lower pole volume is removed to improve parenchymal shaping. De-bulking the lower pole takes stress off the overlying skin and can help maintain shape postoperatively and prevent recurrent ptosis (Fig. 2.40). Be careful not to compromise the "no-go zone" when removing lower pole tissue.

Closure

Deep parenchymal sutures of 2-0 Vicryl are then placed along the vertical incision, bringing the medial and lateral pillars together at the midline (Fig. 2.41).

All incisions are then closed with interrupted 3-0 PDS dermal sutures (Fig. 2.42). The vertical and horizontal scars are closed with a 4-0

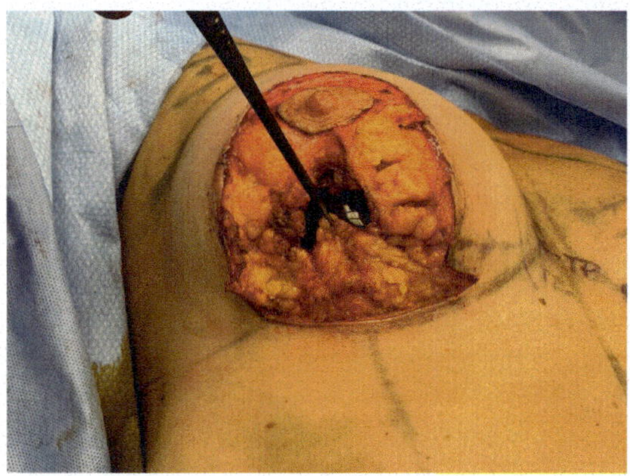

Fig. 2.38 "No-go zone" just above IMF provides an extra layer of protection for the implant

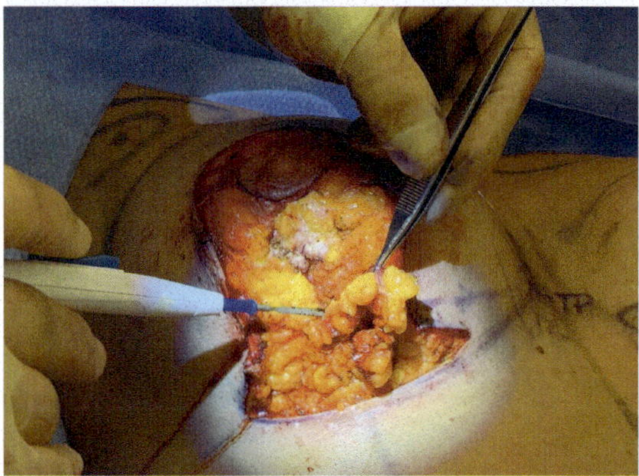

Fig. 2.40 De-bulking of the lower pole after closure of the breast pocket but prior to pillar closure

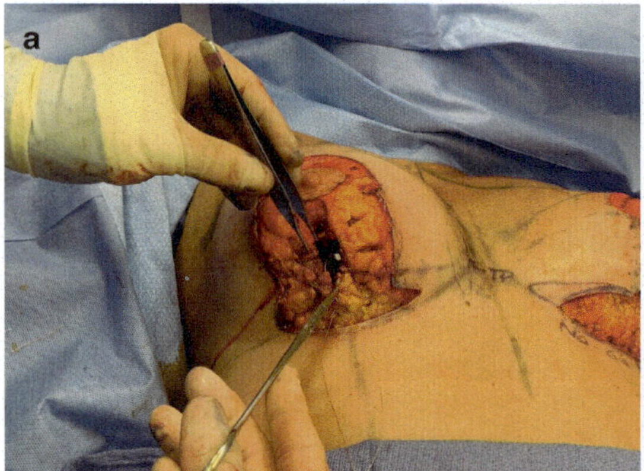

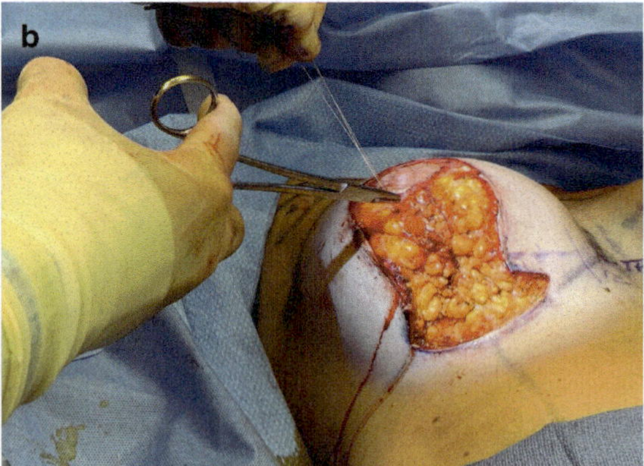

Fig. 2.39 (**a**, **b**) Closure of the posterior lamellae of the implant pocket with a running 2-0 Vicryl suture to provide an additional layer of closure

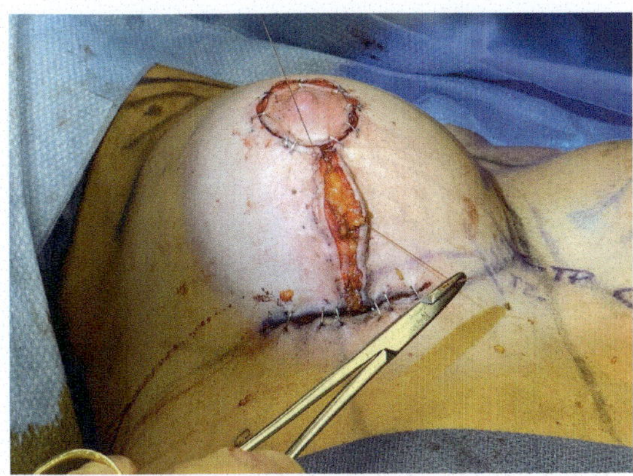

Fig. 2.41 Closure of medial and lateral breast pillars with a 2-0 Vicryl to provide final shape and support of lower breast pole

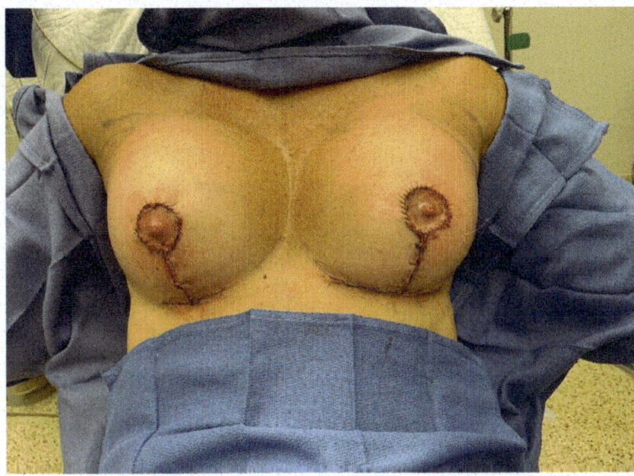

Fig. 2.42 Final closure of the breast with patient sitting upright on the operating room table

Monocryl running subcuticular suture. The areolas are then closed with 3-0 PDS interrupted dermal suture and a simple running 5-0 nylon suture.

Steri-strips are placed over the incision. Contour tape is then placed along the lateral breast border and inframammary fold. The breasts are wrapped with a xeroform gauze, Kerlix, and ace wrap.

Postoperative Care and Expected Outcomes

The patients are instructed to leave all dressing on for 48 hours. The wraps are then removed, and a sports bra is worn for the following 4 weeks. Dressing changes with antibiotic ointment and gauze are used over incisions for 1 week. Patients can shower after 48 hours. The contour tape is removed at day 4–7. Nylons around the areolas are removed 6–7 days postoperatively. The subcuticular Monocryls are clipped on the ends as they exit the skin at 2 weeks. Scar management with silicone gel or silicone sheeting is initiated on all patients at 2 weeks. Patients are allowed to resume activities of daily living almost immediately. Exercise is usually allowed at 4 weeks with heavy lifting at 6 weeks.

Patients are counseled that they can expect swelling and firmness to develop as their breasts heal. The breasts will continue to soften over time, and the breast will relax over the first few months. The results are stable after 6 months, but scars can continue to improve over the first year and some additional relaxation of the breast can continue for even longer.

Complications

The complications in augmentation mastopexy can be considered tissue-related or implant-related [4, 5]. Two separate procedures are being performed and their associated complications are possible. There are very few significant complications in the early postoperative period. The only significant concern early is ischemia to the nipple–areolar complex or skin flaps. Ischemia may be due to the dissection of the pedicle, but often is secondary to excessive tension on the skin closure and underlying volume under the skin flaps. If recognized immediately, all sutures should be removed to evaluate for improved circulation, improved color, adequate capillary refill, and pinprick bleeding. It is important to assure the pedicle is free of tension and not twisted or compromised. Topical nitroglycerin or DMSO (dimethylsulfoxide) can be used to improved venous outflow. If the closure is too tight due to volume present under the flaps, additional breast volume can be removed or the implant downsized/removed in an attempt to reduce the closure tension. If any doubt exists, the wound around the NAC should be left unattached and closed the following day if the NAC has clinically improved.

A hematoma usually occurs within the first 24 hours, but a late hematoma at day 10–14 is also occasionally encountered as activity level increases, and clots are being resorbed at the end of cauterized vessels. Whereas small amounts of blood within the pocket in a mastopexy without a breast implant is generally less concerning, any blood in the breast pocket around an implant requires exploration and a wash out of the pocket to reduce the risk of capsular contracture postoperatively. Early seromas (less than 1 year postoperative) are more often associated with textured implants and often are treated with aspirations alone. If recalcitrant, exchange to a smooth implant may be required.

Secondary Procedures

Late sequelae include poor scarring, recurrent ptosis, implant malposition, asymmetries, late seromas, and capsular contractures. These may require revisional procedures to improve the final aesthetic outcome. Most procedures are delayed at least 6 months or greater to allow for capsule formation, soft tissue remodeling, and stabilization of the results. Scars are often the product of excessive tension on the closure and postoperative swelling and can often be improved with scar revisions when the environment for scar maturation is more optimal. An implant malposition requires internal pocket tightening procedures with possible mesh reinforcement. Lower pole stretch deformities and recurrent ptosis are managed similarly with likely the need for a mastopexy revision.

Capsular contracture is the leading cause of implant-related surgery and can be seen early within the first year or may develop years later. For early capsular contractures, nonoperative measures are initiated including massage (if a smooth implant), ultrasound therapy (Aspen), Vitamin E, Leukotriene-inhibitor (Singulair), and possibly a short course of antibiotics. If nonoperative management fails, surgical intervention is indicated for Grade 3 and 4 capsular contractures. Treatment includes one or more of the following: a capsulectomy, capsulotomy, implant exchange, pocket exchange, placement of acellular dermal matrix, and/or drainage of the breast pocket. In late capsular contractures, it is important to try and solicit any history that may explain its development, such as trauma, dental cleaning, sinus or urinary tract infections, to name a few. In all late capsular contractures, an implant rupture should also be considered. If treatment mandates surgery, the surgeon should be prepared to exchange the implant if ruptured, although the exchange is often planned already to reduce the incidence of recurrence. If treating the capsular contracture nonoperatively, imaging should also be considered to ensure an implant rupture is not present. A late seroma (developing after 1 year) is rare and most associated with textured devices. Although almost always benign, a late seroma is the most common presentation of BIA-ALCL (Breast Implant Associated-Anaplastic Large Cell Lymphoma) and evaluation is mandatory including ultrasound-guided aspiration of the seroma fluid with analysis including testing for CD-30, cell block histology, and flow cytometry. Once BIA-ALCL is ruled out, the seroma can be treated like early seromas. If BIA-ALCL is diagnosed, oncologic surgical intervention should be undertaken.

Conclusion

With proper preoperative evaluation and employing accurate surgical techniques, excellent results can be achieved with an augmentation mastopexy.

Other than the circumareolar approach, all other augmentation mastopexies are approached as vertical mastopexies based on a superior pedicle blood supply. The pedicle selection and design of the procedure do not refer to the skin excisional pattern, which can range from only a vertical scar to a complete inverted-T pattern. In this technique, any pocket and any implant can be used. Avoidance of recurrent ptosis is a hallmark of a successful procedure. Limiting the size of breast implant and aggressively de-bulking the lower pole breast parenchyma minimize this risk. The fascial sling shaping of the lower pole with a lamellar closure over the implant provides additional support and control of breast shape over time. Although considered challenging by most plastic surgeons, mastery of the techniques outlined in this chapter will provide the best framework for optimizing results, minimizing postoperative complications, and ensuring high patient satisfaction.

Case Examples

Case 1 (Fig. 2.43)

Case 2 (Fig. 2.44)

Case 3 (Fig. 2.45)

Case 4 (Fig. 2.46)

Case 5 (Fig. 2.47)

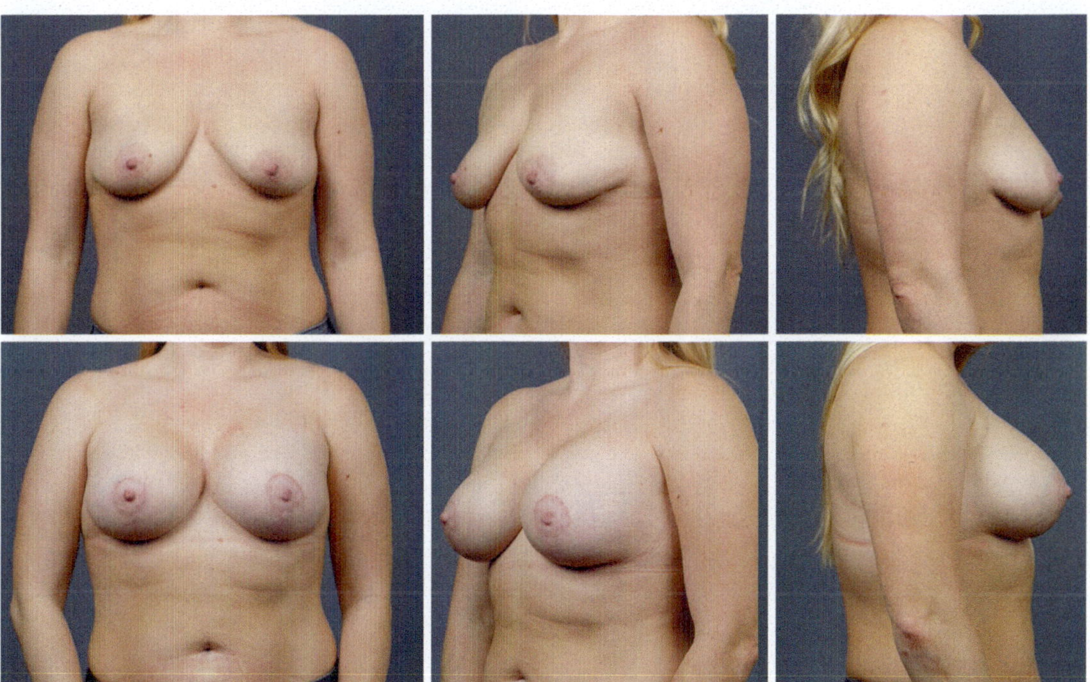

Fig. 2.43 A 33-year-old female with Grade I ptosis. Bilateral periareolar vertical mastopexy with submuscular 350 cc filled to 400 cc on the right and 350 cc filled to 390 cc on the left smooth round moderate plus profile saline implants

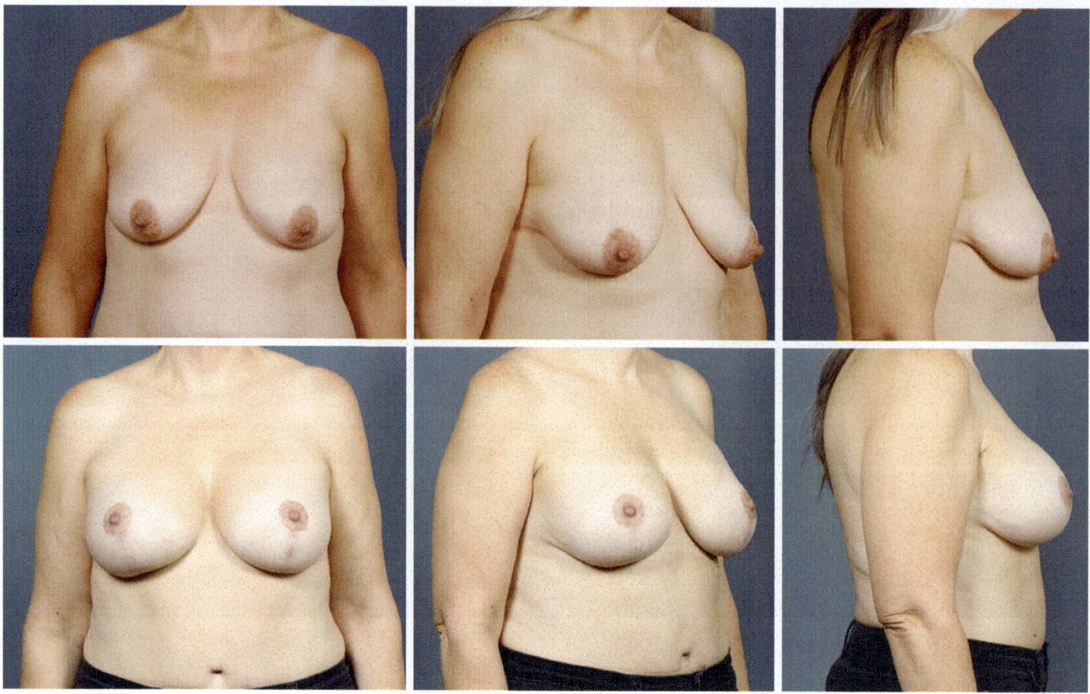

Fig. 2.44 A 54-year-old female with Grade II ptosis. Bilateral full-wise mastopexy with submuscular 425 cc smooth round moderate plus profile silicone implants

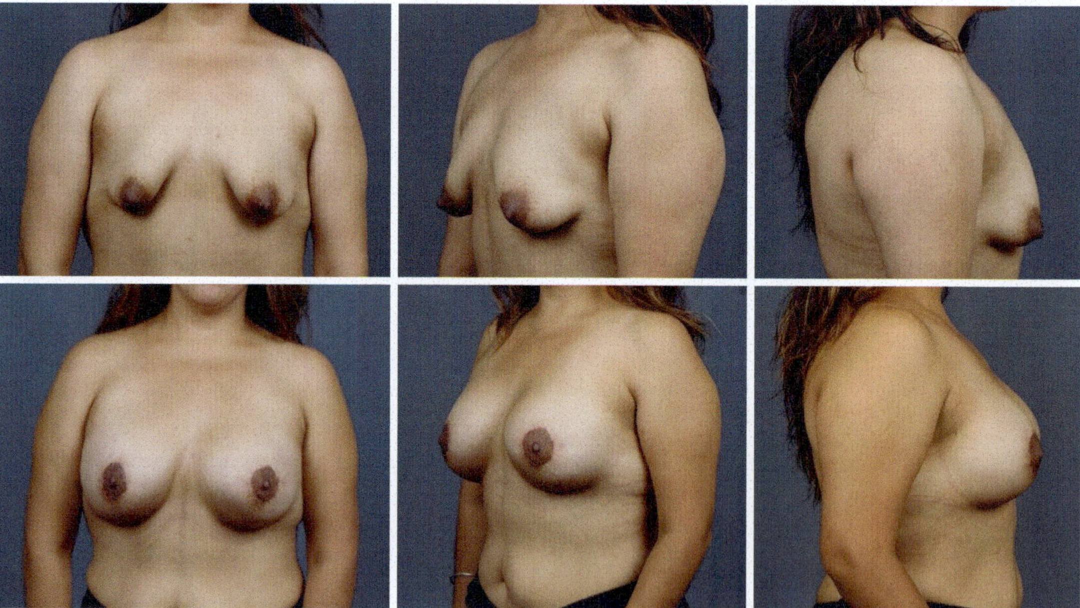

Fig. 2.45 A 27-year-old female with constricted tuberous breast and Grade II ptosis. Bilateral periareolar mastopexy with submuscular dual plane 525 cc on the right and 485 cc on the left textured round moderate profile silicone implants

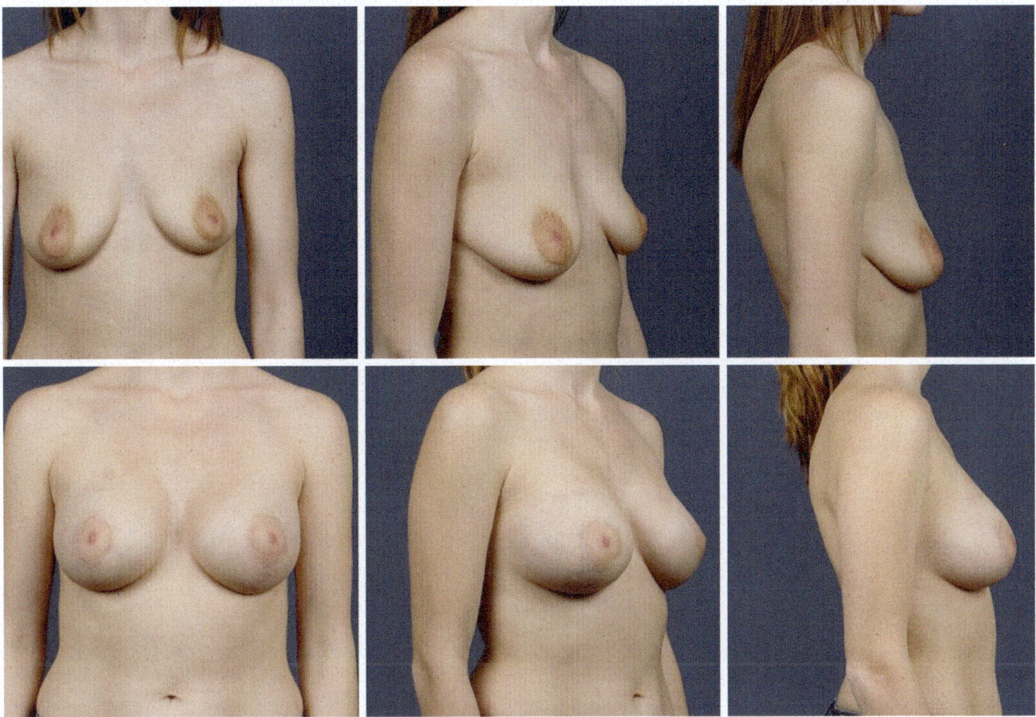

Fig. 2.46 A 24-year-old female with Grade II ptosis. Bilateral periareolar vertical mastopexy with submuscular dual plane 400 cc textured anatomic-shaped moderate profile silicone implants

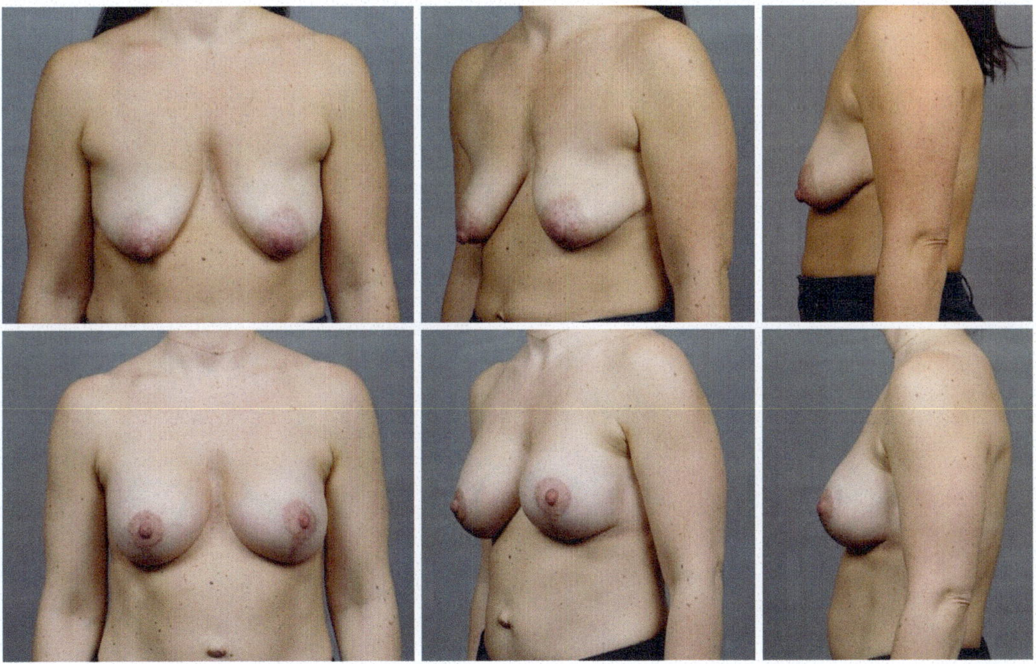

Fig. 2.47 A 40-year-old female with Grade III ptosis. Bilateral periareolar vertical short horizontal mastopexy with submuscular 305 cc smooth moderate profile silicone implants. This patient also underwent bilateral ultrasound-assisted liposuction of the axilla

Editorial Comments This important chapter addresses the hard-to-master treatment of hypoplastic breast in the setting of ptosis. Augmentation mastopexy can be one of the most rewarding but yet frustrating and litigious operation we perform. What makes this operation so challenging are the opposing forces of expansion and tightening that are in play with sometimes less than ideal soft tissue envelope. To strike the right note, the surgeon must have a good understanding of patient's anatomy and tissue quality, biodimensional planning, and mastopexy design.

As the pioneers in this field, Drs. Calobrace and Mays share their expertise with this operation in a detailed and methodical fashion. They review the anatomical features and how they decide between one vs. two stage surgery. It is very important for the novice surgeons to realize that staging is perfectly an acceptable option and sometimes lead to a safer and more superior outcome. The order by which the mastopexy or augmentation is done first will depend on the patient's wish and the degree of ptosis.

The authors highlight some of the differences in biodimensional planning between augmentation and augmentation mastopexy. Importantly, they mention use of lower profile for this operation to minimize waterfall deformity in patients with larger glandular tissue.

The authors do an excellent job of differentiating between the blood supply in a wise pattern breast reduction with inferior pedicle and an inverted-T mastopexy with superior and superomedial pedicle. There are described techniques for preoperative markings for circumvertical and inverted-T mastopexies but they primarily serve an academic purpose and have a less of clinical significance and as the authors point out, the ultimate determination of the design and the amount of skin excision is done with tailor-tacking technique and after the implant is in place.

The authors emphasize the importance of removing some glandular tissue from the lower pole of breast in order to minimize risk of pseudoptosis. It is, however, important to repair the superficial fascia system in this area to help shape the breast just as we repair the SMAS layer in a SMASectomy facelift.

One note of dissent: The authors describe the different ways of accessing the pocket and they primarily use transparenchymal approach such as via the vertical incision for implant placement. Although this may provide some benefit in ease of placing the implant, it exposes the implants to the dreaded breast parenchyma and potentially increases the risk of biofilm formation. In my practice, I use the IMF incision for implant placement regardless of the design for mastopexy. Before ensuing on the mastopexy part, I close the pocket as in primary augmentation. In cases of circumvertical and inverted-T mastopexy I, like the authors, leave a cuff of tissue just above the IMF incision as a security layer to minimize potential implant exposure in case of dehiscence at the T-junction.

Congratulations again to Drs. Calobrace and Mays for their excellent chapter on augmentation mastopexy.

Kiya Movassaghi

References

1. Hoffman S. Some thoughts on augmentation/mastopexy and medical malpractice. Plast Reconstr Surg. 2004;113:1892–3.
2. Nahai F, Fisher J, Maxwell GP, Mills DC II. Augmentation mastopexy: to stage or not. Aesthet Surg J. 2007;27:297–305.
3. Spears SL. Augmentation mastopexy: "surgeon beware". Plast Reconstr Surg. 2003;112:905–6.
4. Stevens WG, Macias LH, Spring M, Stoker DA, Chacón CO, et al. One-stage augmentation mastopexy: a review of 1192 simultaneous augmentation and mastopexy procedures in 615 consecutive cases. Aesthet Surg J. 2014;34:723–32.
5. Calobrace MB, Herdt DR, Cothron KJ. Simultaneous augmentation/mastopexy: a retrospective 5-year review of 332 consecutive cases. Plast Reconstr Surg. 2013;131:145–56.
6. Tessone A, Millet E, Weissman O, Stavrou D, Nardini G, Liran A, et al. Evading a surgical pitfall: Mastopexy-augmentation made simple. Aesthet Plast Surg. 2011;35:1073–8.
7. Lee MR, Unger JG, Adams WP. The tissue-based triad: a process approach to augmentation mastopexy. Plast Reconstr Surg. 2014;134:215–25.
8. Persoff MM. Mastopexy with expansion-augmentation. Aesthet Surg J. 2003;23:34–9.
9. Binelli L. A new periareolar mammoplasty: the "round block" technique. Aesthet Plast Surg. 1990;14:93–100.
10. Lejour M. Vertical mammoplasty for breast reduction and mastopexy. In: Spear SL, editor. Surgery of the breast: principles and art. Philadelphia: Lippincott-Raven; 1998. p. 73.
11. Hall-Findlay EJ. Pedicles in vertical breast reduction and mastopexy. Clin Plast Surg. 2002;29:379–91.
12. Wise RJ. Treatment of breast hypertrophy. Clin Plast Surg. 1976;3:289–300.
13. Marchac D, Olarte G. Reduction mammoplasty and correction of ptosis with a short inframammary scar. Plast Reconstr Surg. 1982;69:45–55.
14. Tebbetts JB. Form stability of the style 410 implant: definitions, conjectures, and the rest of the story. Plast Reconstr Surg. 2011;128:825–6.
15. Calobrace MB, Capizzi PJ. The biology and evolution of cohesive gel and shaped silicone implants. Plast Reconstr Surg. 2014;134(1S):6S–11S.
16. Regnault P. Breast ptosis. Definition and treatment. Clin Plast Surg. 1976;3:193–203.
17. Hall-Findlay EJ. Applied anatomy: key concepts for modern breast surgery. In: Hall-Findlay EJ, editor. Aesthetic breast surgery: concepts and techniques. St. Louis: Quality Medical Publishing, Inc.; 2011.
18. Kalaaji A, Dreyer S, Brinkmann J, Maric I, Nordahl C, Olafsen K. Quality of life after breast enlargement with implants versis augmentation mastopexy: a comparative study. Aesthet Surg J. 2018;38(12):1304–15.

19. Tebbetts JB, Teitelbaum S. High- and extra-high-projection breast implants: potential consequences for patients. Plast Reconstr Surg. 2010;126(6):2150–9.
20. Namnoun JD, Largent J, Kaplan HM, Oefelein MG, Brown MH. Primary breast augmentation clinical trial outcomes stratified by surgical incision, anatomical placement and implant device type. J Plast Reconstr Aesthet Surg. 2013;66:1165–72.
21. Calobrace MB, Stevens WG, Capizzi PJ, Maric I, Nordahl C, Olafsen K. Risk factor analysis for capsular contracture: a 10-year Sientra study using round, smooth, and textured implants for breast augmentation. Plast Reconstr Surg. 2018;141(4S):20S–8S.
22. Hall-Findlay EJ. Breast implant complication review: double capsules and late seromas. Plast Reconstr Surg. 2011;127:56–66.
23. Spear SL, Rottman SJ, Glicksman C, Brown M, Al-Attar A. Late seromas after breast implants: theory and practice. Plast Reconstr Surg. 2012;130(2):423–35.
24. Loch-Wilkinson AL, Beath KJ, Knight RJW, Wessels WLF, Magnusson M, Papadopoulos T, et al. Breast implant-associated anaplastic large cell lymphoma in Australia and New Zealand: high surface-area textured implants are associated with increased risk. Plast Reconstr Surg. 2017;140(4):645–54.
25. Tebbetts JB. Dual plane breast augmentation: optimizing implant-soft-tissue relationships in a wide range of breast types. Plast Reconstr Surg. 2012;130(2):423–35.
26. Regnault P, Daniel RK, Tirkanits B. The minus-plus mastopexy. Clin Plast Surg. 1988;15:595–600.
27. Spring MA, Macias LH, Nadeau M, Stevens WG. Secondary augmentation-mastopexy: indications, preferred practices, and the treatment of complications. Aesthet Surg J. 2014;34(7):1018–40.
28. Flugstad NA, Pozner JN, Baxter RA, Creasman C, Egrari S, Martin S, et al. Does implant insertion with a funnel decrease capsular contracture? A preliminary report. Aesthet Surg J. 2016;36:550–6.
29. Mladick RA. "No-touch" submuscular saline breast augmentation technique. Aesthet Plast Surg. 1993;17:183–92.

3 Shaping the Breast: Composite Breast Augmentation

James M. Smartt Jr and Louis P. Bucky

Introduction

Over the last 15 years, the process of breast augmentation has been guided by the concept of biodimensional planning, in which an implant works in harmony with the surrounding soft tissue envelope to provide optimal aesthetic results. Generally speaking, the processes of implant selection and its three-dimensional placement have dominated the process, with numerous well-established approaches to implant selection in patients with highly variable presentations in chest wall shape, breast location and size, and associated soft tissue coverage [1]. As traditional planning for breast augmentation has been restricted to implant selection, the results of breast augmentation are sometimes limited to the variability of the implants themselves and to a lesser degree the associated incisions or method of access to the breast pocket. The process of composite breast augmentation removes many of these limitations by altering the breast's soft tissue envelope itself—thereby providing a more versatile technique to locate and manipulate the composition of the breast mound. As a result, the breast implants and fat "work together" and provide the best qualities of each: the core volume projection of implants combined with the desired softness and natural behavior of fat. Moreover, fat grafting to the periphery of the breast can actually change the dimensions of the natural breast, thus allowing for more options in implant selection. The technique is also particularly useful in revision cases such as capsular contracture or rippling with associated implant visibility. Furthermore, when combined with an associated mastopexy to alter the position of the nipple–areolar complex, the process of composite breast augmentation is incredibly versatile and provides superior results in a wide range of patients.

J. M. Smartt Jr (✉) · L. P. Bucky
Bucky Plastic Surgery, Ardmore, PA, USA
e-mail: smartt@drbucky.com

Composite Breast Augmentation

The term "composite breast augmentation" refers to the placement of a breast prosthesis for core volume with the addition of variable amounts of autologous fat in the surrounding soft tissue envelope. With the advent of autologous fat grafting to the breast, surgeons gained a useful tool to optimize implant/soft tissue relationships in a wide variety of patients. Fat grafting to the breast has become an integral piece of the breast surgeon's armamentarium—with increasing enthusiasm following the reversal of the American Society of Plastic Surgeon's reversal of its moratorium on the process in 2008. Since then, the technique has been used by a number of surgeons with generally excellent results [2–6]. The versatility of the technique has much to do with the characteristic of fat itself. Adipose tissue is a readily available autologous substance that can be harvested with

K. Movassaghi (ed.), *Shaping the Breast*, https://doi.org/10.1007/978-3-030-59777-1_3

minimal morbidity and placed in precise locations and in variable volumes. Once donor fat is vascularized in its new location, the tissue is soft and behaves in ways analogous to native breast tissue.

To understand the role of the breast prosthesis in composite breast augmentation, one might start by asking the following question: Why it is not optimal to treat every patient that seeks breast enlargement with fat grafting alone? As fat grafting to the breast gains increasing acceptance, and many patients have adequate donor tissue, why would anyone want to incur the risks associated with breast implants? In our experience, it is critical to understand the role of the implant in creating *core volume* and *projection*. Increases in core volume, or the deep centrally located portion of the breast mound, are difficult to attain using autologous fat for a variety of reasons. One, the central portion of the breast mound tends to be increasingly glandular, especially in younger patients, and this denser breast tissue is generally not an optimal recipient environment for autologous fat. Furthermore, while it is not technically impossible to introduce into the central portion of the breast, the number of grafting sessions that would be required to create similar increases in volume would likely prove prohibitive. Simply put, an appropriately sized breast implant is the most cost-effective and timely way to provide sufficient core breast volume. Furthermore, many patients seeking breast augmentation desire some form of enhancement of the superior pole of the breast—a change that can only be provided by altering the overall projection of the breast mound. In many cases, autologous fat grafting alone is insufficient to provide appreciable changes in projection. While fat grafting can provide increases in volume, this enlargement tends to result in a fusiform increase in size with similar contour to the preoperative state, especially in the upper pole of the breast. For this reason, when patients seek enhancement in the upper pole of the breast, we generally recommend either conventional breast augmentation or composite breast augmentation using an appropriately sized breast implant.

The role of fat grafting in composite breast augmentation is, therefore, *generally limited to changes in the periphery of the breast and the superficial soft tissue envelope.* The authors stress that the utility of this technique should not be underappreciated. Given the vast majority of implant-related complications are not due to the performance of the device, per se, but instead to the quality of the surrounding soft tissue, the utility of composite breast augmentation becomes increasingly apparent. Examples of common soft tissue problems that can be treated include (but are not limited to) the following:

- Deficiency of soft tissue in the medial breast with insufficient cleavage and a lateral bias of the breast mound
- Excessively thin portions of the overlying soft tissue envelope with associated rippling or implant visibility
- Poorly located breast prostheses with associated discontinuity of the surrounding soft tissue envelope, that is, double-bubble deformities

Before discussing particular cases in which composite breast augmentation might be useful, let us first revisit common methods employed using the technique.

Surgical Technique

The authors tend to avoid rigid typologies when discussing the technique of composite breast augmentation. In so much as a wide range of patients that can be adequately treated using the method, composite breast augmentation is truly a versatile technique applicable to a variety of situations in both primary and secondary breast augmentation and breast reconstruction. Nonetheless, the individual techniques used in the approach are fairly reproducible.

Fat Harvest/Liposuction

For the vast majority of our cases, we employ an "in-line" collection system. The flanks, lateral thighs, and abdomen are generally the fat harvest sites. These sites undergo superwet tumescent infiltration with roughly 1:1 volumes of tumescent solution to lipoaspirate. In the majority of cases, a total of 200–500 cc of lipoaspirate is harvested using a 3-mm multiport liposuction cannula. The harvested fat is placed into 50-cc syringes and undergoes manual centrifugation for 2 minutes.

Breast Implant Placement

The authors recognize that the landscape surrounding breast implantation is rapidly changing. Given these concerns, the authors have moved almost entirely to the use of smooth variably cohesive gel implants. While there are many settings in which the use of textured implants had advantages in the hands of many providers, it is worth noting that again, composite augmentation renders many of these advantages irrelevant as the surrounding soft tissue envelope can be manipulated to a greater degree. The thickness of the subcutaneous plane between skin and prosthesis can be increased by the addition of fat, thus providing coverage for all implant types. In nearly all cases, implant placement is performed in the subpectoral plane (dual plane 1) via a 4-cm inframammary incision. In primary augmentations, the device is placed via the aid of a Keller funnel. In general, implant selection is consistent with the overall concept of biodimensional planning. It is noteworthy to recognize some of the implications of composite breast augmentation for implant selection. It has been widely recognized that suboptimal results in conventional breast augmentation are oftentimes the result of "asking the implant to do too much." This commonly occurs in the setting of a breast prosthesis that is at the upper ranges of recommended size and results in the characteristic soft tissue attenuation. What follows, unfortunately, is a predictable cascade of soft tissue attenuation, resulting in downstream effects such as implant palpability, visibility or rippling, and possible capsular contracture. Composite breast augmentation largely removes the pressure on the surgeon to sometimes place implants at the upper limit of recommended size or beyond. Instead, fat grafting reinforces the soft tissue envelope (and provides for additional volume) with autologous fat—especially in areas where soft tissue attenuation can be particularly problematic, that is, the medial and lateral breast margins in thinner patients.

Fat Grafting in Primary Breast Augmentation

The particular method of fat grafting is generally determined by the demands of the particular patient, but the preparation of the fat and its delivery mechanisms are fairly universal. Grafting is performed using 50-cc syringes affixed with 15-cm long 1.5-mm blunt-tipped fat grafting cannulas (Byron Medical Inc.). This form of cannula is generally optimal as retrograde placement of the fat can be performed with good efficiency. The cannula is relatively blunt which is important as the glide plane between implant capsules and the subcutaneous tissue can be reliably located without undue implant trauma. Grafting itself should be performed in the methods advocated by Coleman and others—depositing small aliquots of fat in multiple areas within a particular tissue plane, all the while avoiding the creation of "lakes" or excessively large individual grafts.

In terms of fat grafting volumes, there are some basic guidelines we find helpful. Fat grafting is generally performed in reproducible locations with volumes that fall within predictable ranges. Other authors have provided theoretical estimates of the volumes of fat that would be required to attain specified increases in soft tissue thickness [3]. These estimates can be useful when performing subtotal coverage of a breast implant. In the author's experience, such cases are not very common. The vast majority of patients undergoing composite breast augmentation receive treatment to select areas of the breast that require soft tissue modification. One common situation in primary augmentation is the thin patient whose medial breast is deficient in soft tissue (Fig. 3.1). In situations such as these, we have generally found that grafting 25–150 cc (with an average of roughly 100 cc) of autologous fat on the medial aspects of each breast is sufficient to provide adequate soft tissue coverage in this area. As these patients have generally not experienced any of the iatrogenic effects of prior surgery, the grafting requirements are generally modest [5]. The judicious use of fat grafting, while respecting the concept of "graft to recipient site ratio," rarely leads to fat necrosis or cyst formation in these patients. Although no one knows this exact ratio, it is certainly less than 1:1.

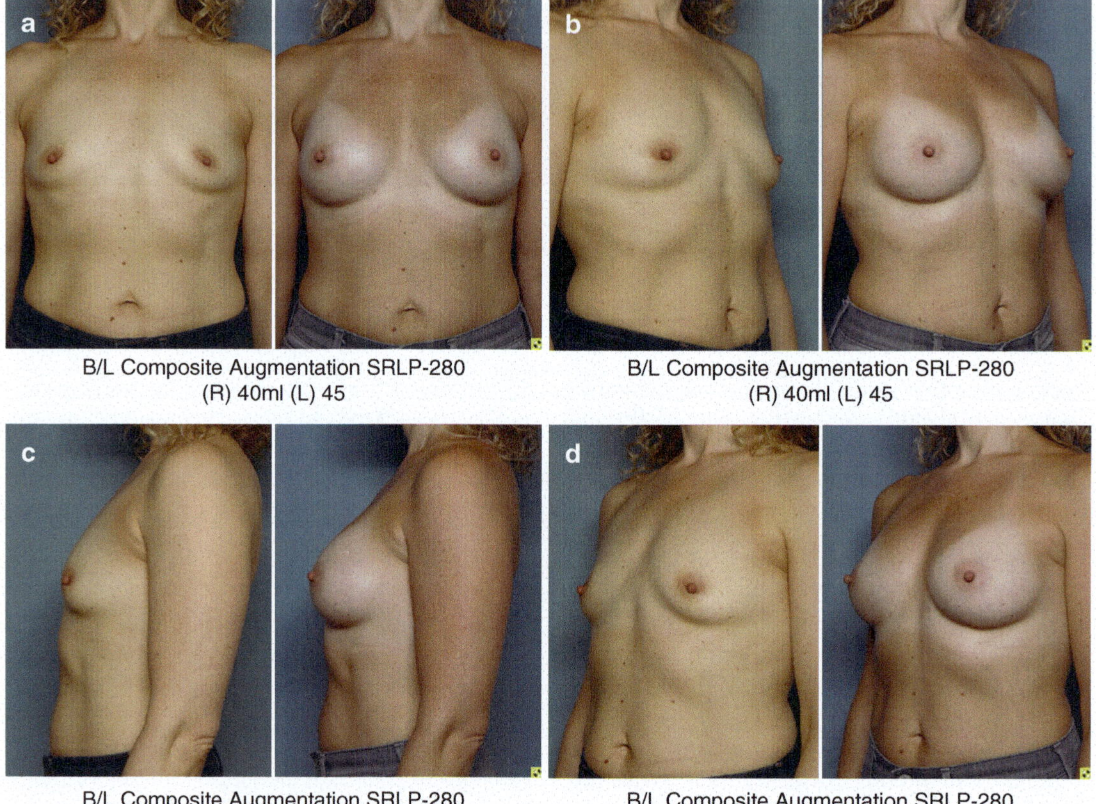

Fig. 3.1 (**a–e**) Primary composite breast augmentation. (Left) Preoperative photos. The patient demonstrates anatomic characteristics that are regarded as challenging in the setting of conventional breast augmentation: a deficiency of parenchymal tissue, lateral placement of the breast mound, and insufficient medial soft tissue coverage. Bilateral breast augmentation was performed using 280 cc smooth round cohesive gel moderate profile silicone implants. The prosthesis was placed in the submuscular plane via an inframammary incision. Simultaneously, fat grafting was performed along the medial aspects of both breasts to provide for sufficient cleavage and to reduce the likelihood of implant visibility; 40 cc of fat was grafted to the right breast and 45 cc to the left. Fat grafting was performed in the subcutaneous plane. (Right) Postoperative photos. Note the well-contoured result with medialization of the breast mound and appropriate soft tissue fullness of the medial breast

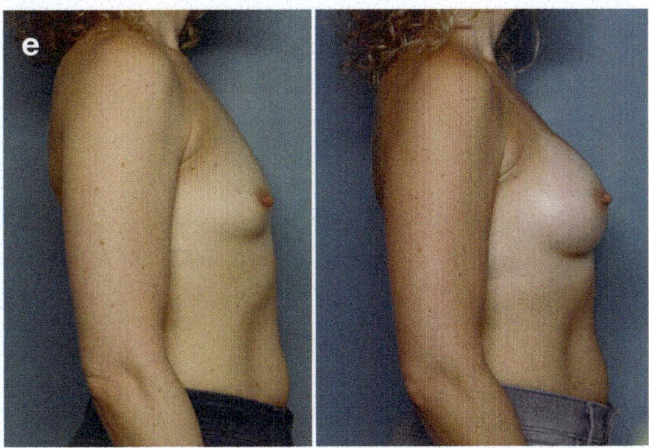

B/L Composite Augmentation SRLP-280
(R) 40ml (L) 45

Fig. 3.1 (continued)

Fat Grafting in Secondary Breast Augmentation

Secondary augmentation and secondary breast reconstruction have more similarities than differences. Frequently, more donor tissue can be required to create the desired soft tissue improvement. In these cases, the surgeon faces a soft tissue envelope of an entirely different composition. In addition, techniques like needle band release and capsule preservation are as important as fat placement in these situations. The factors that may have contributed to the patient's preoperative state are myriad—scarring from prior surgery, capsule formation, iatrogenic soft tissue attenuation, and the presence of an implant are all factors that must be considered when planning revision surgery. In these challenging cases, it is common to want to provide a global improvement in soft tissue coverage. Sometimes these cases can require multiple rounds of fat grafting to attain the desired result. Generally, to provide total anterior coverage of an existing implant the authors would graft each breast with a range of 100–300 cc of fat per breast, with the vast majority of secondary cases requiring roughly 150 cc to 200 cc per side (Fig. 3.2). As the volumes of fat increase, so does the likelihood of complications related to grafting, including fat necrosis, cyst formation, and graft failure. In addition, grafting in a more hostile environment should lead to conservative volumes. Given that many of the patients in this category are relatively thin individuals with insufficient soft tissue coverage in the first place, it stands to reason that multiple rounds of fat grafting may be required as donor site adipose tissue can sometimes be challenging to harvest.

Needle Band Release

Needle band release is a versatile technique that often accompanies secondary composite breast augmentation. It is important to first discuss the role that needle band release, or the creation of small vascularized potential spaces, plays in appropriate fat grafting of the breast. Mere injection of autologous fat into the younger adult or previously operated breast can be challenging. Graft take is greatly affected by the quality of the vascular network in which the fat is grafted. Ideally, autologous fat will have the best "take" if micro-aliquots of fat are placed within well-vascularized spaces. These spaces should still maintain a controlled (albeit small) domain. Using the technique of needle band release, the constricting elements of a variety of breast deformities can be adequately treated. This technique provides for additional volume without the creation of large devascularized spaces or "lakes" with poor graft take and the increased likelihood of complications like fat necrosis and cyst formation. Examples of primary cases where needle band release is particularly useful include challenges such as the tuberous breast or constricted breast [7–10].

The authors have found that the technique of needle band release (NBR) provides for the creation of increased surface area and appropriately shaped and vascularized potential spaces in which to then graft autologous fat. A description of the technique is provided below. In the author's experience, fat grafting combined with NBR can enhance the shape by removing or releasing certain constrictions related to both iatrogenic and congenital deformities. An example of using the NBR technique would include releasing the constricting ring associated with

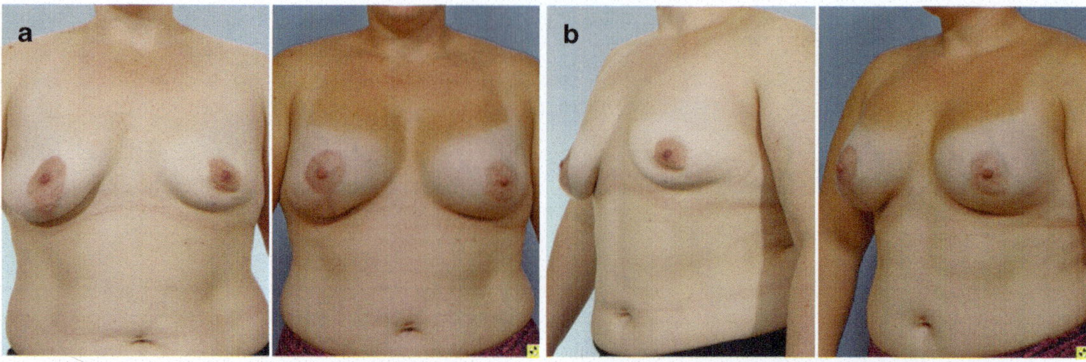

H/O Previous Breast Augmentation; Deflated Saline Implants.
B/L R/R of Breast Implants (R)SRM-405 (L) SRM-445;
Right Vertical Wedge Mastopexy; LVFG to B/L Breast (R) 95ml (L) 130

H/O Previous Breast Augmentation; Deflated Saline Implants.
B/L R/R of Breast Implants (R)SRM-405 (L) SRM-445;
Right Vertical Wedge Mastopexy; LVFG to B/L Breast (R) 95ml (L) 130

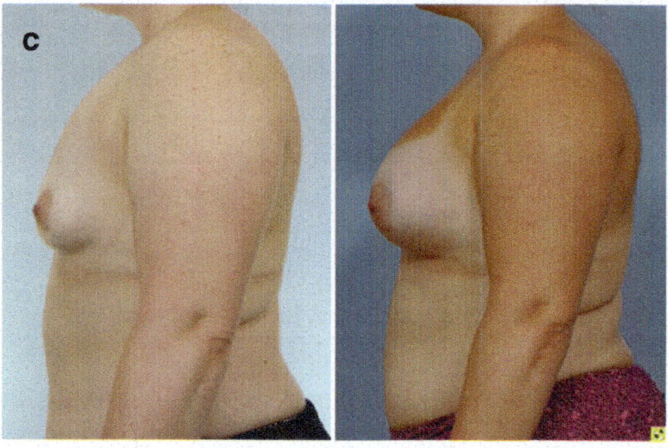

H/O Previous Breast Augmentation; Deflated Saline Implants.
B/L R/R of Breast Implants (R)SRM-405 (L) SRM-445;
Right Vertical Wedge Mastopexy; LVFG to B/L Breast (R) 95ml (L) 130

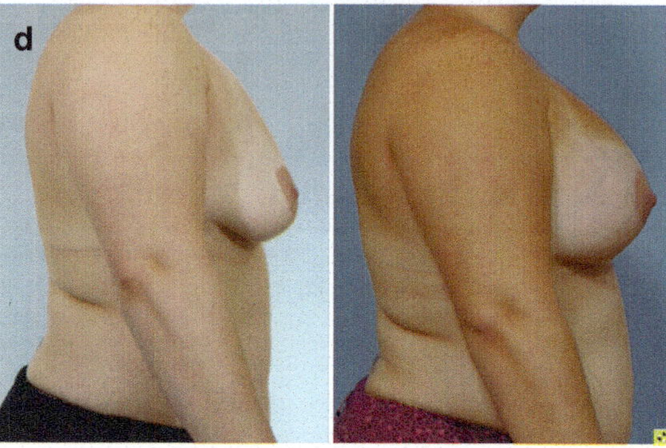

H/O Previous Breast Augmentation; Deflated Saline Implants.
B/L R/R of Breast Implants (R)SRM-405 (L) SRM-445;
Right Vertical Wedge Mastopexy; LVFG to B/L Breast (R) 95ml (L) 130

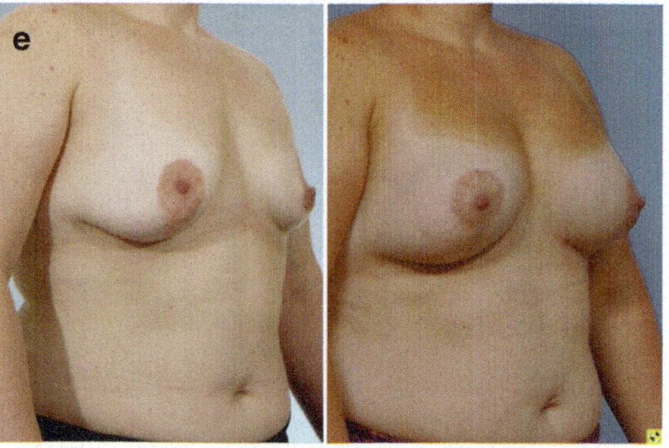

H/O Previous Breast Augmentation; Deflated Saline Implants.
B/L R/R of Breast Implants (R)SRM-405 (L) SRM-445;
Right Vertical Wedge Mastopexy; LVFG to B/L Breast (R) 95ml (L) 130

Fig. 3.2 (**a**–**e**) Secondary composite breast augmentation and mastopexy. (Left) Preoperative photos. This particular patient had a history of previous breast augmentation with saline implants. These devices were deflated in the office prior to removal and replacement of the implants with composite breast augmentation and balancing mastopexy. Preoperative deflation of the previous breast implants allows the creation of a potential space in which to place autologous fat. In this particular case, 95 cc of fat was grafted to the right breast and 130 cc to the left breast. This was performed during one session of grafting simultaneously with implant exchange. (Right) Postoperative photos. This example is illustrative of how the technique can be useful in the setting of prior surgery and diverse patient presentations. Of note, this degree of projection of the superior pole of the implants is likely not attainable with fat grafting alone. The appearance of the breasts is globally improved with corresponding improvement in the thickness of the soft tissue coverage of the replaced silicone breast implants

the areolar deformity in the tubular breast, or the ripples associated with attenuated soft tissue coverage and capsular contracture.

Patient Examples

Primary Composite Breast Augmentation

This case is illustrative of a common clinical problem: thinner patients that are at a high risk of implant visibility and lateralization of the breast mound following traditional breast augmentation (see Fig. 3.1). Generally, these patients are fairly thin and present with significant hypomastia and a preexisting lateral bias of the nipple–areolar complex. In the context of traditional biodimensional planning, it would be difficult to achieve appropriate cleavage or a smooth appearance of the medial breast.

Surgical Technique

In the senior author's experience, we prefer smooth round silicone gel implants. A modestly sized prosthesis is placed in the subpectoral plane via a 4 cm inframammary incision. Minimal release of the sternal portions of the pectoralis major muscle is performed (dual plane 1). Fat grafting is performed following the harvest of donor tissue from the flanks, thighs, or abdomen. Grafting takes place after insertion of the prosthesis and closure of the Scarpa's fascia. Nearly all of the grafting is performed in the subcutaneous plane and all of the graft volume is placed along the medial aspects of the breast via the inframammary incision. Signs of volume limits of grafting include peaux de orange, free flow of fat out the incisions, tightness of the soft tissue envelope, and lack of resistance when passing the cannula [11].

Revision Composite Breast Augmentation

These cases are quite diverse in their presentation and sometimes require variable graft volumes to attain the desired results. In this particular example, the patient has undergone prior breast augmentation (see Fig. 3.2). Following deflation of the prostheses preoperatively, a significant potential space is created to accept a significant volume of graft material. Deflation of the prostheses also exposes significant preexisting breast asymmetry that will require a concomitant mastopexy to attain the desired correction. In this case, again a moderately sized smooth gel implant is chosen.

Surgical Technique

Deflation of the exiting prostheses takes place in the office under local anesthesia. One month following deflation, composite augmentation mastopexy is performed. In these cases, the sequence of fat grating can vary as the existing capsule is a well-vascularized tissue plane that can support significant volumes of grafting. Moreover, it protects against grafting into the potential space created by the implant. This offers a stable host bed that is anatomically different from the subcutaneous plane. In many instances, this capsular plane is an excellent first pass during the grafting procedure and can be performed prior to insertion of the revision implant. If further grafting is needed, this can also be performed in the subcutaneous plane. In cases such as this, needle band release is sometimes quite helpful in providing directed expansion of specific quadrants of the breast. The technique is often particularly useful in preferential expansion of a constricted inferior pole, or in areas of rippling and capsular contracture where there is inadequate space between the implant and overlying skin. Granted, in these cases serial grafting may be required. Implant placement is universally performed via an inframammary incision. However, it can be performed remotely from a transaxillary approach, as well. Prior to composite breast augmentation, a wide variety of techniques would be performed to manipulate or reinforce the existing capsule in order to optimize the position of the breast mound. Utilizing composite breast augmentation, suboptimal characteristics of the breast mound can be independently addressed with fat grafting. Furthermore, grafting can be performed in a staged fashion to address a wide variety of deformities of the breast.

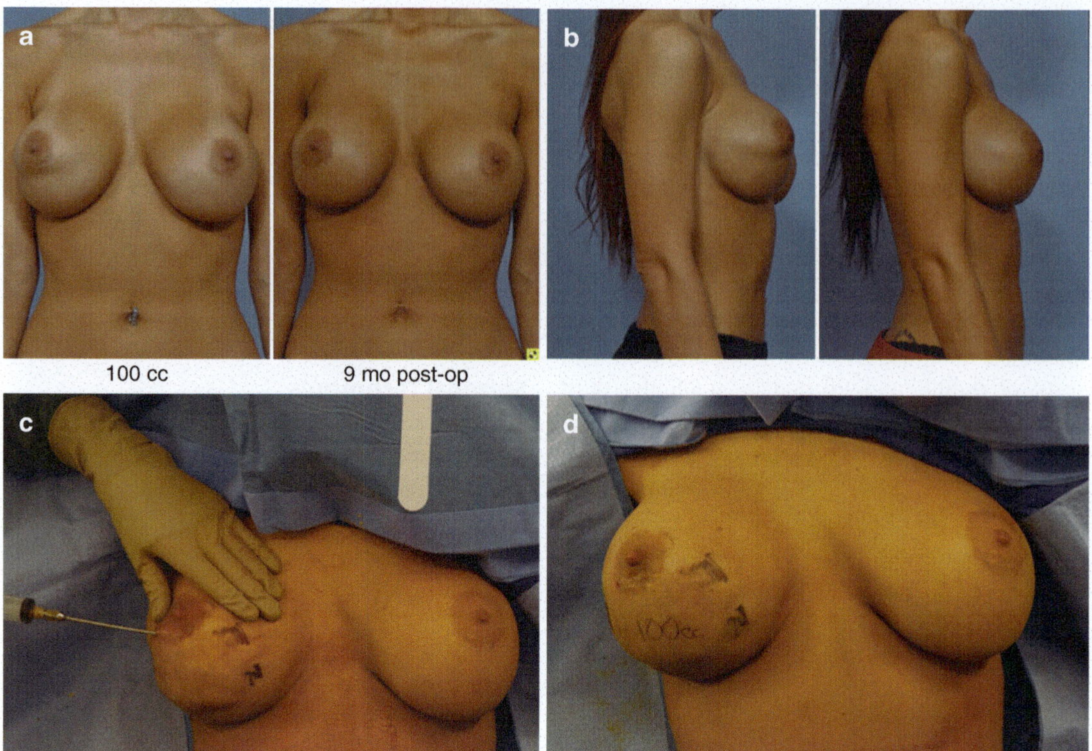

Fig. 3.3 (**a–d**) Secondary composite breast augmentation for treatment of double-bubble deformity. (Left) Preoperative photos. (Right) Postoperative photos at 9 months following fat grafting. This patient demonstrates the attenuation of the soft tissue envelope of the inferior pole of the right breast that is associated with the double bubble deformity. The patient underwent grafting of 100 cc of autologous fat via a periareolar stab incision. Grafting is performed in the subcutaneous plane using a 15-cm long 1.5-mm blunt-tipped fat grafting cannula. This procedure can reliably be performed by grafting on top of the existing implant capsule and any remaining subcutaneous space. Note that following placement of the graft there is appropriate overcorrection of the defect. This patient required only one session of fat grafting to provide appropriate soft tissue coverage

Another common indication for the use of composite breast augmentation is the "double bubble" deformity. In these cases, the inferior pole of the breast generally becomes deficient in soft tissue coverage with resulting visibility of the inferior pole of the implant (Fig. 3.3). In these cases, the soft tissue envelope of the inferior pole of the breast can be markedly attenuated—sometimes with associated misplacement of the inframammary crease. Prior to the use of autologous fat grafting, the operative solution for these cases would sometimes involve complex soft tissue rearrangement, relocation of the implant to another tissue plane, with possible replacement of the prosthesis itself. All of these maneuvers entailed significant operative risk and a prolonged recovery. In the era of composite breast augmentation, the double bubble deformity can be treated with autologous grafting. This treatment entails significantly less operative risk. Even in cases of severe soft tissue attenuation, grafting can be performed safely in the subcutaneous plane and directly on top of the existing implant capsule.

Conclusion

Composite breast augmentation is a versatile technique. The favorable characteristics of breast implants and autologous fat can be combined to attain superior results in both primary and secondary breast augmentation.

Editorial Comments Fat injection is changing the landscape in many areas of plastic surgery, and I believe we are still scratching the surface. In this chapter, Drs. Smartt and Bucky provide an excellent overview of the role of fat injection in breast surgery while making sure that the readers understand its limitations and potential complications as we push the envelope. Just like other procedures, it is not meant to be the "holy grail" but rather an adjunct to other techniques in breast surgery.

I agree with the authors that fat injection can only be used to improve the periphery of the breast envelope. Any effort to use fat injection to increase breast conus will be disappointing and can increase complication rates, that is, fat necrosis.

As we have moved away from textured implants more recently, we are seeing a rise in implant-related complications. Many of these complications are due to the unfavorable relationship between implants and surrounding soft tissue envelope (e.g., uncontrolled tissue expansion, which I described in Chap. 1). This is especially prevalent with the larger implants with eventual soft tissue attenuation. As the authors indicated, fat injection in composite augmentation provides the added benefit of reducing the mechanical stress of the implant by allowing one to choose a smaller implant and augment it with autologous fat. They also list other indications for fat to correct many of the secondary issues.

One small note of dissent: Although placement of implants in the submuscular pockets, which is the authors' preference, may provide some advantages, such as increased sensitivity of mammograms and less visibility, it can also introduce its own risk of animation deformity, pistol effect, and weakness, to name a few. Over time, my approach with many surgeries has become more "holistic"; hence, I use the subfascial pocket much more often. Traditionally, we have used the 2 cm thickness of the upper pole as a threshold to decide between prepectoral and subpectoral augmentation. Now, with better cohesive implant options, use of smaller implants and fat injection to the periphery of the breast, many more women are candidates for prepectoral augmentation with much less morbidity.

Congratulations again to the authors for their excellent chapter. I would especially like to thank Dr. Bucky, who became my role model in my early years of training as I used to watch him perform complex reconstructive surgery at Massachusetts General Hospital.

Kiya Movassaghi

References

1. Tebbetts JB. Dual plane breast augmentation: optimizing implant-soft-tissue relationships in a wide range of breast types. Plast Reconstr Surg. 2006;118(7 Suppl):81S–98S; discussion 99S–102S.
2. Auclair E, Anavekar N. Combined use of implant and fat grafting for breast augmentation. Clin Plast Surg. 2015;42(3):307–14, vii.
3. Auclair E, Blondeel P, Del Vecchio DA. Composite breast augmentation: soft-tissue planning using implants and fat. Plast Reconstr Surg. 2013;132(3):558–68.
4. Kerfant N, Henry A-S, Hu W, Marchac A, Auclair E, et al. Subfascial primary breast augmentation with fat grafting: a review of 156 cases. Plast Reconstr Surg. 2017;139(5):1080e–5e.
5. Bravo FG. Parasternal infiltration composite breast augmentation. Plast Reconstr Surg. 2015;135(4):1010–8.
6. Maione L, Caviggioli F, Vinci V, Lisa A, Barbera F, Siliprandi M, et al. Fat graft in composite breast augmentation with round implants: a new concept for breast reshaping. Aesthet Plast Surg. 2018;42(6):1465–71.
7. Brault N, Stivala A, Guillier D, Moris V, Revol M, François C, et al. Correction of tuberous breast deformity: a retrospective study comparing lipofilling versus breast implant augmentation. J Plast Reconstr Aesthet Surg. 2017;70(5):585–95.
8. Claudio Silva-Vergara C, Fontdevila J, Weshahy O. Fat grafting technique, a paradigm shift in the treatment of tuberous breast. World J Plast Surg. 2018;7(1):72–7.
9. Delay E, Sinna R, Ho Quoc C. Tuberous breast correction by fat grafting. Aesthet Surg J. 2013;33(4):522–8.
10. Derder M, Whitaker IS, Boudana D, Marchac A, Hivelin M, Mattar N, et al. The use of lipofilling to treat congenital hypoplastic breast anomalies: preliminary experiences. Ann Plast Surg. 2014;73(4):371–7.
11. Del Vecchio DA, Bucky LP. Breast augmentation using preexpansion and autologous fat transplantation: a clinical radiographic study. Plast Reconstr Surg. 2011;127(6):2441–50.

4 Shaping the Breast: Optimizing Aesthetics with Reconstructive Breast Surgery

Maurice Y. Nahabedian

Introduction

Reconstructive breast surgery has now entered the realm of aesthetic breast surgery. No longer is it acceptable to merely create just a breast mound following mastectomy because current expectations are to reconstruct a breast that mimics the natural form and, in some cases, even exceeds it. The reasons for this are multifactorial, but ultimately the result of a variety of innovations and advancements that have resulted in our ability to achieve surgical and aesthetic outcomes that were not possible 20 years ago. This is true for reconstruction with prosthetic devices, autologous tissues, and oncoplasty.

The concept of the "bio-engineered breast" applies not only to prosthetic reconstruction but also to autologous reconstruction because both of these options offer the potential to create a beautifully shaped and contoured breast [1]. Common to autologous and prosthetic reconstruction has been nipple-sparing mastectomy. As nipple-sparing mastectomy has been the focus and desire of many women having therapeutic or prophylactic mastectomy, breast surgeons have optimized their surgical technique and pay more attention to issues related to vascularity of the mastectomy skin flaps and make all attempts to preserve the normal subcutaneous fat of the breast. This results in an optimal mastectomy skin envelope that will enhance reconstructive and aesthetic outcomes. The other advancement that is useful for autologous and prosthetic reconstruction is fat grafting. Fat grafting has been demonstrated to improve breast contour and skin quality following autologous and prosthetic reconstruction and has been especially useful following radiation therapy.

Specific to prosthetic reconstruction has been the use of acellular dermal matrices, highly cohesive breast implants, and prepectoral placement of prosthetic devices. Specific to autologous reconstruction is the use of perforator-based flaps that completely spares the donor site muscles. We now practice in an era of muscle preservation that includes the rectus abdominis muscle with DIEP flaps and the pectoralis major muscle with prepectoral reconstruction.

This chapter provides an update on surgical techniques and strategies for autologous, prosthetic, and oncoplastic breast reconstruction that have improved outcomes for patients following total or partial mastectomy.

Prosthetic Reconstruction

Prosthetic breast reconstruction is the most common form of reconstruction offered to women with breast cancer. Procedural statistics from the American Society of Plastic Surgeons

M. Y. Nahabedian (✉)
Department of Plastic Surgery, Virginia Commonwealth University – Inova Branch, McLean, VA, USA

K. Movassaghi (ed.), *Shaping the Breast*, https://doi.org/10.1007/978-3-030-59777-1_4

demonstrate that of the 106,295 breast reconstructions performed in 2017, 84,979 were with prosthetic devices (79.9%) and 19,316 were with autologous flaps (20.1%) [2]. This trend toward increasing prosthetic reconstruction is occurring at a rate of 11%/year whereas autologous reconstruction rates have remained flat [3, 4]. The increase is multifactorial and due to increasing rates of contralateral prophylactic mastectomy (15%/year) and bilateral prophylactic mastectomy (12%/year). Other factors include the use of acellular dermal matrices, autologous fat grafting, and nipple-sparing mastectomy. All of these factors have improved the quality of prosthetic breast reconstruction and have contributed to the increase.

The challenge for prosthetic based reconstruction is to achieve predictability and reproducibility so that aesthetic outcomes are optimized and complications are minimized [5–7]. In order to achieve these goals, surgeons must consider several factors related to appropriate patient selection and operative technique. Proper patient selection is based on appreciating the likelihood of an adverse event based on body mass index (BMI), prior radiation, mammary hypertrophy, tobacco use, poorly controlled diabetes mellitus, etc. Operative technique includes the use of acellular dermal matrices, degree of pectoralis major coverage, autologous fat grafting, and whether the reconstruction is performed in one or two stages. This chapter reviews many of these factors and provides a framework to optimize outcomes and minimize complications.

Patient Selection

The importance of proper patient selection cannot be overemphasized [8]. Patient selection begins at the initial consultation by obtaining a thorough history and physical examination that includes comorbidities, tobacco history, body habitus, and breast characteristics. The occurrence of adverse events can be directly attributed to a variety of factors including elevated BMI (>40), active tobacco use, and poorly controlled diabetes mellitus. Mammary hypertrophy in and of itself is not a contraindication to prosthetic breast reconstruction; however, there are several strategies that can increase the likelihood of a successful outcome. Most women with mammary hypertrophy will have large mastectomy skin excision patterns because traditional skin or nipple sparing is usually not an option. The two common mastectomy incisions in these patients include the inverted T incision and the extended transverse/oblique skin excision pattern [9–11]. With both methods, the goal is to adequately reduce the skin envelope to fit the initial phase of the prosthetic reconstruction. The two-stage technique is preferred in women with severe mammary hypertrophy in order to better define an optimal breast contour. Secondary contouring procedures are often necessary in women with mammary hypertrophy.

Device Selection

Selection of the appropriate devices for prosthetic breast reconstruction requires clinical examination and breast measurements. The most important measurement is the base width of the breast that will assist with the selection of a tissue expander or implant. Tissue expanders are uniformly designed and include a contoured shape, textured surface, suture tabs, and an integrated port. Permanent implant selection is based on breast measurements, tissue compliance, and patient expectations. In a two-stage implant-based reconstruction, the tissue expander width is selected a little narrower than the final implant for better pocket control. Breast implants vary in terms of size (100–800 cc), filler material (saline or silicone gel), surface (smooth or textured), and shape (round or anatomic). The majority of patients and surgeons prefer silicone gel implants because they mimic the natural breast more closely. Shaped breast implants tend to be more form stable and maintain the natural slope of the upper pole with less rippling and wrinkling. Round implants are commonly used because they tend to be softer than shaped devices and move more like a natural breast.

Immediate Versus Delayed Reconstruction

The decision to proceed with immediate versus delayed reconstruction is complex and requires considerable attention. Factors that may influence this decision are based on the stage of the cancer, advanced patient age, obesity, patient comorbidities, tobacco use, prior radiation therapy, and technical aspects related to the mastectomy. There are demographic data to suggest that immediate breast reconstruction is increasing at the rate of 5%/year [3, 4]. Benefits of immediate reconstruction include improved aesthetic outcomes, less psychological stress, and the convenience of completing the mastectomy and reconstruction at the same time. Disadvantages of immediate reconstruction include an increased rate of adverse events such as mastectomy skin flap necrosis and the potential to interfere with adjuvant treatments compared to delayed reconstruction.

It has been estimated that mastectomy skin flap necrosis occurs in 5–30% of patients following immediate breast reconstruction [12–15]. Strategies to minimize mastectomy skin flap necrosis include preservation of the subcutaneous fat and subdermal vascular plexus as well as the internal mammary perforating vessels following mastectomy. When skin flap perfusion is in question, fluorescent angiography has been advocated to assess tissue perfusion immediately following mastectomy and has been demonstrated to reduce the incidence of mastectomy skin flap necrosis from 15.1% to 4% [16]. Nitroglycerine ointment has also been demonstrated to improve local circulation when perfusion has been compromised [17]. When mastectomy skin flap perfusion is compromised, the technique of delayed–immediate reconstruction by closing the mastectomy defect without reconstruction and returning at a later date to initiate the reconstructive process has demonstrated success [18].

Acellular Dermal Matrix

The use of acellular dermal matrix (ADM) is commonly used for partial subpectoral and prepectoral prosthetic breast reconstruction [19–21]. The benefits include added tissue support, prevention of window-shading with contraction of the pectoralis major, reduction in periprosthetic scar formation, compartmentalization of the prosthetic device, and improved definition of the infra-mammary and lateral-mammary folds. Figures 4.1 and 4.2 illustrate the use of ADM for partial subpectoral and prepectoral reconstruction, respectively. Although used by many plastic surgeons, controversy regarding its use remains. In two systematic reviews comparing total and partial muscle coverage with and without ADM, the complication profile was similar between the two cohorts [22–24].

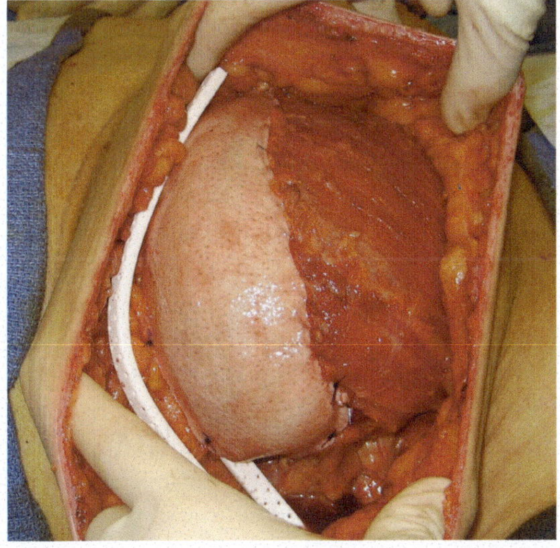

Fig. 4.1 Dual-plane prosthetic reconstruction utilizing ADM

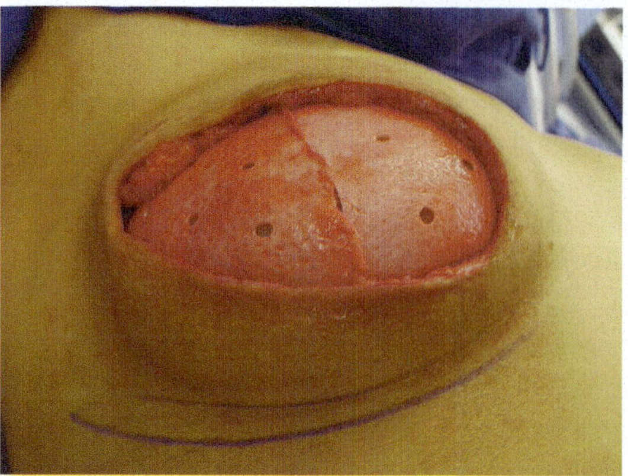

Fig. 4.2 Prepectoral prosthetic breast reconstruction utilizing ADM

Partial Subpectoral Prosthetic Breast Reconstruction and ADM

Partial subpectoral placement of a device involves incising the inferior origin of the pectoralis major muscle and elevating the muscle off of the chest wall. Acellular dermal matrices are used as an extender to secure the inferior edge of the pectoralis major muscle to prevent window-shading or excessive cephalad migration of the muscle (see Fig. 4.1). This approach can be used in the setting of one- or two-stage breast reconstruction. The surgical technique is similar for both and the outcomes and aesthetic quality of the reconstruction can be excellent. As with all elements of breast reconstruction, optimizing aesthetics will depend on proper patient selection and surgical technique [25, 26]. The decision to proceed with one-stage (direct-to-implant) reconstruction will depend on the quality of the mastectomy skin flaps in terms of thickness and perfusion. Direct-to-implant reconstruction can be performed with skin- or nipple-sparing mastectomy [27, 28]. It is important to assess tissue perfusion using clinical judgment and fluorescent angiography [16]. Device selection is based on bio-dimensional planning to ensure that the footprint of the implant correlates with the footprint of the mastectomy space. Round or shaped implants can be used and are based on the desired contour and projection of the breast (Figs. 4.3 and 4.4).

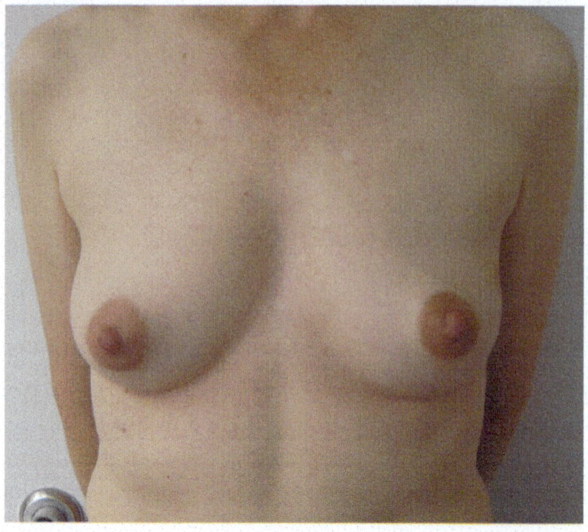

Fig. 4.3 Preoperative photograph of a woman with left breast cancer

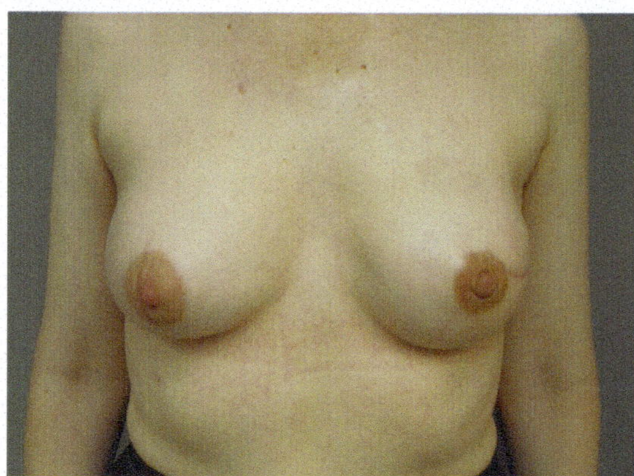

Fig. 4.4 Postoperative image following left nipple-sparing mastectomy and direct to implant reconstruction with contralateral augmentation for symmetry

The two-stage technique will also deliver excellent aesthetic outcomes and is considered by many surgeons to be more predictable. Two-stage reconstruction is usually recommended in women with mammary hypertrophy, when mastectomy skin flaps may not tolerate direct-to-implant reconstruction, or surgeon preference [29, 30]. The technical aspects of placing a tissue expander are similar to that of placing an implant with the primary difference being that the tissue expanders are usually tabbed which allows them to be sutured to the chest wall. The use of ADM is similar for one- or two-stage reconstruction. The tissue expander is usually partially filled, thus offloading pressure on the mastectomy skin flaps and theoretically reducing the likelihood of mastectomy skin flap necrosis. Following complete expansion and completion of adjuvant therapies, the second stage is planned. This occurs no sooner than 3 months following the initial insertion of the tissue expander to allow enough time for ADM adherence and adequate stress relaxation of the skin. If the capsule is thick, a capsulotomy is performed as needed. If the capsule is thin and there is lateral or inferior migration of the device, a capsulorrhaphy is performed. A round implant is usually selected when upper pole considerations are low and the patient desires a soft breast. A shaped silicone gel implant is selected when there is a need to optimally contour the upper pole. Autologous fat grafting can be considered at this stage to additionally fill the upper pole, to increase the thickness of the mastectomy skin flaps, and to improve the quality of the soft tissues. Figures 4.5 and 4.6 illustrate a patient following two-stage, dual-plane, prosthetic breast reconstruction.

Prepectoral Prosthetic Breast Reconstruction

Prepectoral placement has become a preferred approach for many plastic surgeons [6, 7, 11, 19, 20, 31, 32]. The benefits of prepectoral placement include elimination of animation deformities, less postoperative pain, no spasm of the pectoralis major muscle, and more natural breast aesthetics. Breast aesthetics are usually enhanced with prepectoral because the medial origin of the pectoralis major does not impede optimal placement of the implant. The requirements for prepectoral placement include well-vascularized mastectomy skin flaps with appropriate thickness (no visible dermis). Many plastic surgeons consider the use of an ADM a prerequisite for prepectoral reconstruction to provide additional soft tissue support and to provide stability to the prosthetic device. Prepectoral device placement can be performed in the setting of skin-sparing or nipple-sparing mastectomy as well as one- or two-stage reconstruction.

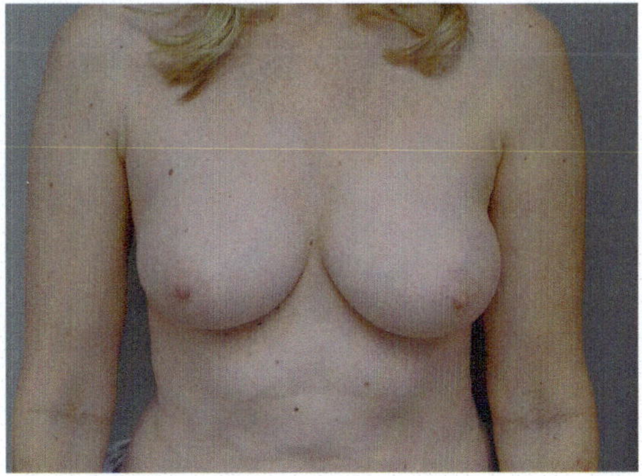

Fig. 4.5 Preoperative photograph of a woman with the BRCA mutation

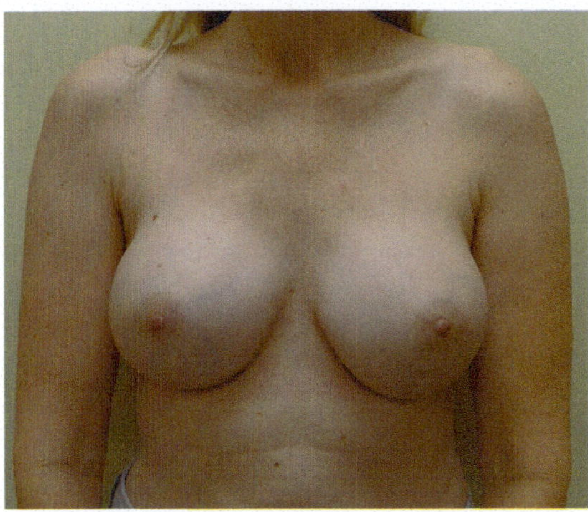

Fig. 4.6 Postoperative photograph following bilateral nipple-sparing mastectomy and two-stage prosthetic reconstruction

One of the caveats with prepectoral breast reconstruction (prosthetic devices and flaps) is the possibility of obscuring tumor detection (via palpation) when it is near the chest wall. This has always been a concern with autologous reconstruction placed above the pectoralis major muscle and is now a concern with prosthetic devices placed above the pectoralis major muscle. For this reason, practitioners often recommend avoiding immediate prepectoral reconstruction following mastectomy when the breast cancer is within 5 mm of the pectoralis major muscle. Fortunately, this represents the minority of patients so prepectoral reconstruction can be safely performed in the vast majority of patients. In patients who are at moderate-to-high risk for chest wall recurrence who have had a reconstruction above the pectoralis, MRI following reconstruction is recommended to assess for tumor recurrence.

Following confirmation of skin flap perfusion, the decision to proceed with one- or two-stage reconstruction is made. The technique of ADM use is varied. A single large sheet 16 × 20 cm or two smaller sheets (16 × 6 or 16 × 8 cm) can be used [33]. The ADM can be wrapped around the device and sutured posteriorly along the undersurface of the device with spanning sutures (off-label technique) or the ADM can be sutured directly to the outlined pattern of the prosthetic device on the pectoralis major muscle (on-label technique). With one-stage reconstruction, it is important to achieve a snug hand-in-glove fit between the ADM and the prosthetic device to minimize the risk of implant rotation or migration. Implant selection can include round or shaped devices based on the desired aesthetic goals of the operation (Figs. 4.7 and 4.8). With the two-stage technique, the tissue expander is sutured to the chest wall to provide stability. Closed suction drains are required to create a negative pressure within the periprosthetic space, to facilitate adherence of the ADM to the mastectomy skin, and to reduce the incidence of seroma. Once expansion is complete, the second stage is planned. During this stage, the tissue expander is exchanged for a permanent implant and autologous fat grafting is performed as needed (Figs. 4.9 and 4.10). The fat grafting will reduce the likelihood of rippling and wrinkling and can optimally contour the breast. Fat grafting is typically performed using 1- to

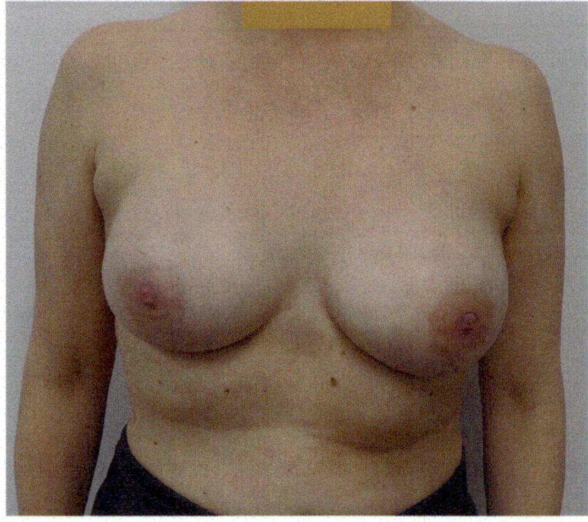

Fig. 4.8 Postoperative photograph following bilateral nipple-sparing mastectomy and direct to implant breast reconstruction

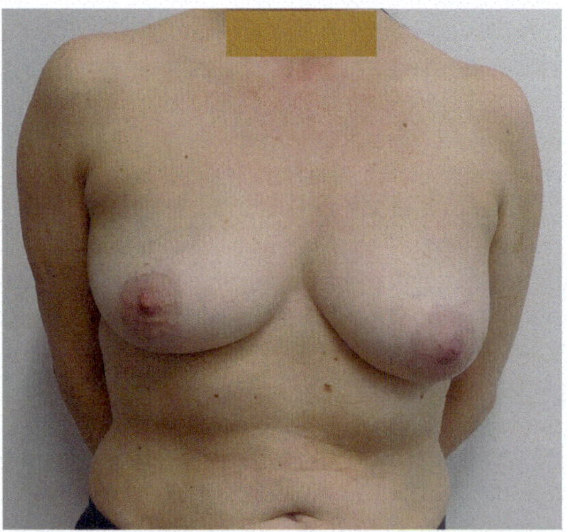

Fig. 4.7 Preoperative photograph of a woman with right breast cancer

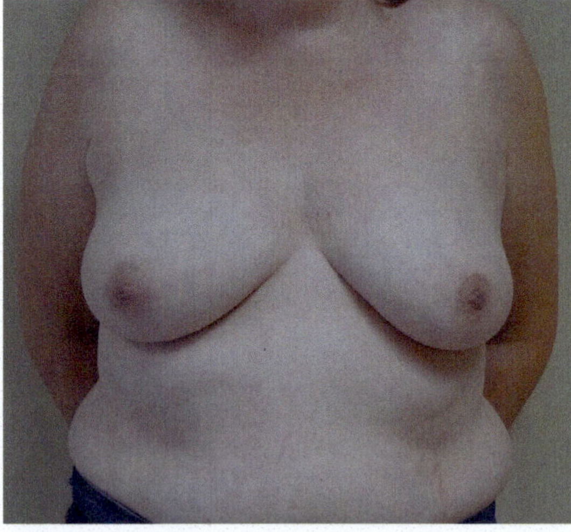

Fig. 4.9 Preoperative photograph of a woman with right breast cancer

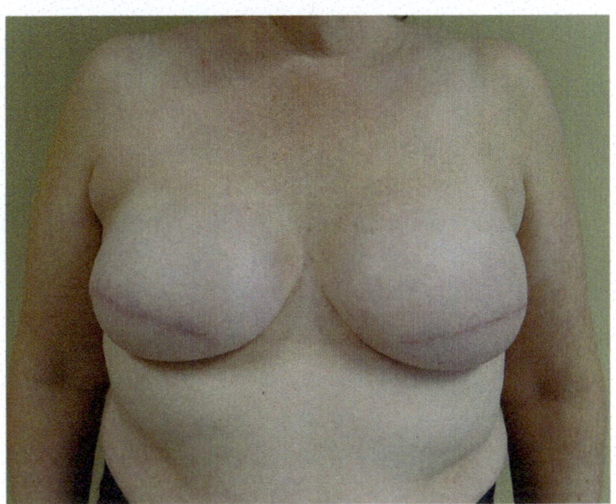

Fig. 4.10 Postoperative photography following bilateral skin-sparing mastectomy and two-stage prosthetic breast reconstruction

2-mm cannulas inserted into the subcutaneous layer between the skin and the ADM. Typical fat volumes range from 75 to 200 cc based on breast size and dimensions.

Autologous Fat Grafting and Prosthetic Breast Reconstruction

Autologous fat grafting has been a significant advancement in the setting of prosthetic breast reconstruction to improve surgical outcomes. Its safety profile in women with a history of breast cancer and reconstruction has been demonstrated in several studies [34–36]. Kaoutzanis et al. have demonstrated that fat grafting after breast reconstruction resulted in a biopsy rate of 7.4% and no cases of locoregional cancer recurrence [34]. Seth et al. demonstrated that fat grafting after breast reconstruction did not adversely affect local tumor recurrence or survival on long-term follow-up [35]. The efficacy of autologous fat grafting has been demonstrated based on an improvement in breast contour and tissue quality primarily via the role of stem cells [36].

Complications from fat grafting include fat necrosis, oil cysts, microcalcifications, poor retention, infection, palpable nodules, and contour abnormalities [37, 38]. Minimizing complications requires a fundamental understanding of the nature and process of fat grafting. Fat is a metabolically active and heterogeneous tissue consisting cytokines, hormones, and various growth factors. Every step with autologous fat grafting is important and includes the harvesting, processing, and transplantation process. The critical element is the viability of the fat and stem cells prior to transplantation. The specifics related to the technique and details of fat grafting are beyond the scope of this chapter and the readers are encouraged to read additional references [39, 40].

Techniques to improve the likelihood of success with fat grafting are related to fat preparation, timing, and recipient site preparation. Studies have demonstrated that fat viability is retained despite differences in processing or harvesting techniques [39]. Fat retention after fat grafting for breast reconstruction is dependent on time and volume [40]. Its efficacy in radiated and non-radiated patients has been observed, as retention volume was independent of previous radiation or the site of fat harvest. Studies have demonstrated that fat retention can be improved by adequate preparation of the recipient site. The technique of percutaneous aponeurectomy is especially important to release the fibrous bands within the recipient site [41]. This allows for optimal lipofilling without the increased resistance to injection that can decrease fat cell viability especially in previously radiated tissues.

Radiation Therapy and Prosthetic Breast Reconstruction

Radiation therapy is known to increase rates of reoperation, reconstructive failure, and total complications in the setting of prosthetic breast reconstruction [42, 43]. The adverse events include capsular contracture, infection, delayed healing, incisional dehiscence, premature removal of device, and asymmetry. In a review of 146 women following breast reconstruction and radiation therapy, Nahabedian demonstrated removal of prosthetic device in 23 of 52 women (44%). Of these, 45% were removed when radiation followed breast reconstruction and 43%

were removed when radiation preceded breast reconstruction [43]. In another review of 100 consecutive patients following prosthetic breast reconstruction, the complication rate was 44% when radiation was delivered prior to reconstruction, 23% when radiation was delivered following device reconstruction, and 11.7% in the setting of no radiation [44]. Specific complications included infection, seroma, and incisional dehiscence.

Capsular contracture is known to occur with greater frequency following radiation therapy. Seruya et al., in a review of 336 ADM-assisted prosthetic breast reconstructions following dual-plane reconstruction, demonstrated a significant increase in the rate of capsular contracture when comparing radiated to non-radiated breasts (29.6% vs. 0.7%) at a mean follow-up of 16.1 months [45]. An interesting observation with prepectoral prosthetic breast reconstruction is that the classic appearance of cephalad migration of the prosthetic device in the setting of partial subpectoral placement is not observed [46, 47]. It is postulated that the radiation-induced contracture of the pectoralis major muscle promotes the cephalad displacement of the devices.

Improving outcomes in the setting of prosthetic reconstruction and radiation therapy is challenging. The timing of radiation therapy relative to prosthetic reconstruction has been studied. Cordeiro et al. have compared patients having radiation therapy in the setting of tissue expanders ($n = 94$) or permanent implants ($n = 210$) and demonstrated that reconstructive failure occurred in 32% tissue expanders and 16.4% of implants at 6 years suggesting that tissue expander to implant exchange occurring prior to radiation is associated with less reconstructive failure [48]. Within the same cohorts, grade 3 and 4 capsular contracture occurred in 17.1% of patients with radiated tissue expanders and in 50.9% of patients with radiated implants demonstrating the discrepancy. In a similar study, Nava demonstrated a reconstructive failure rate of 6% when radiation was delivered to the permanent implant and 40% when delivered to the tissue expander [49]. Reasons for failure included capsular contracture, infection, and device exposure.

Autologous Reconstruction

Many surgeons and patients consider the use of autologous tissue for breast reconstruction to represent the gold standard. This is because autologous breast reconstruction represents the use of one's own tissue, will last forever, and often improves over time. The use of prosthetic devices is usually not necessary but can be used to augment the reconstruction. A variety of flaps from various donor sites have been described that have provided women with excellent outcomes and a high quality of life [50–63]. The most commonly utilized donor sites are from the abdomen and include the transverse rectus abdominis musculocutaneous (TRAM), deep inferior epigastric perforator (DIEP), and superficial inferior epigastric artery flaps (SIEA). Other flaps include the latissimus dorsi musculocutaneous and thoracodorsal artery perforator flaps (TDAP), inferior and superior gluteal artery perforator flaps (IGAP, SGAP), and the transverse upper gracillis (TUG) and profunda artery perforator flaps (PAP).

It is important to have an appreciation of ideal breast aesthetics when considering autologous reconstruction. The position of the breast on the chest wall should serve as footprint for the breast to be reconstructed. The natural shape or cone of the breast should be appreciated in order to estimate the amount of skin that will be required to achieve ideal proportions. It is important to understand the relationship of the torso to the breast in order to reconstruct a breast that will be appropriate for the patient's frame and body habitus. The ultimate goal is to create symmetry, proportion, and contour.

The three-step principalization of breast reconstruction described by Phillip Blondeel is an excellent strategy to achieve ideal breast aesthetics and is based on the breast footprint, the conus, and the skin envelope [64–67]. The footprint is unique for each woman and defined and fixed for each breast. The borders of the footprint include the clavicle, lateral edge of the sternum, anterior axillary line, and the inframammary fold. The footprint represents the foundation for the conus. The conus represents the three-dimensional shape, volume, projection, and contour of the breast. In general, ideal breast proportions are based on the upper-pole to lower-pole ratio and defined as 45:55 [68]. The final component is the skin envelope. In the setting of immediate reconstruction, the quality and quantity of skin is important and affected by previous surgery, radiation, scar, and vascularity.

Patient Selection

Proper patient selection and successful surgical outcomes are intimately related [8]. Although many women interested in breast reconstruction following mastectomy may be candidates for autologous reconstruction, not all may be. Candidacy may be precluded for reasons such as medical comorbidities, extremes of body habitus, prior operative procedures at the donor site, or a desire for a quick and simple procedure.

When evaluating women for autologous breast reconstruction, several factors should be considered that are related to specific characteristics of the patient and breast. These include breast volume and contour, body habitus, donor site considerations, medical comorbidities, tumor characteristics, patient preference, and the need for adjuvant therapies. The abdomen has been the donor site of choice for most women and requires a sufficient quantity of fat in order to create a desired breast with sufficient vascularity. Prior operations at a particular donor site may preclude the use of that flap because of the risk of damage to the angiosomes, perforators, or source vessels. Although a woman may be slender with a paucity of fat, she may still be a candidate for autologous reconstruction if the breast volume requirements are low. In women who are overweight or obese, a flap can still be performed; however, the flap should be tailored to sustain its perfusion requirement and to minimize the incidence of fat necrosis as well as partial flap necrosis.

Patients should also be evaluated for comorbidities prior to proceeding with autologous reconstruction. Specific comorbidities or factors that may preclude immediate autologous reconstruction include active tobacco use, poorly controlled diabetes mellitus, cardiac disease, and hypercoaguable states. Patients are advised to stop using tobacco products for 4 weeks prior to surgery and for 2 weeks postoperatively. Diabetic patients should maintain strict glucose control and maintain a hemoglobin A1c level less than 7 to avoid problems with healing. Hypercoaguable states should be recognized preoperatively to avoid thrombotic events that can result in microvascular failures. Obese patients with a body mass index exceeding 40 are usually advised to lose weight to minimize the incidence of adverse events. Performing breast reconstruction in obese patients is not a contraindication; however, patients must be aware that complications such as delayed healing, infection, and flap failure may be slightly increased. Proper patient selection is a prerequisite to reduce complications and improve aesthetic outcomes.

The topic of complications is discussed and reviewed with all women [69–71]. Common complications to all flaps include total flap failure, partial flap failure, fat necrosis, and delayed healing. Total flap failure rates are generally less than 2%. Fat necrosis may occur in 0–10% of cases. The incidence of infection and hematoma are generally low and range from 0% to 3%. Other morbidities are more specific to the donor site. Abdominal flaps may be prone to weakness depending on the degree of muscle trauma or sacrifice. A bulge or hernia can also occur and ranges from 0% to 10%. Latissimus dorsi flaps are prone to seroma formation that occurs in 5–25% of patients. Gluteal flaps may be prone to seroma formation, contour irregularities, and pain. Thigh-based flaps may be complicated by complex scars or lymphedema.

Flap Selection

Flap selection is ultimately based on the volume requirements of the new breast and donor site availability. The abdomen is the most commonly used donor site with its many varieties that include the pedicle TRAM, free TRAM, DIEP, and the SIEA flap. When the abdomen is not suitable the secondary donor sites are typically considered that include the posterior thorax, gluteal, and thigh regions. The various flaps will be reviewed.

Abdominal Flaps

Inherent to the understanding of abdominal flaps is an appreciation to the amount of muscle that is elevated with the flap [70]. Flap classification is based on the amount of rectus abdominis preserved on the abdominal wall. The rectus abdominis muscle can be separated into three longitudinal segments: medial, lateral, and central. The MS-0 (muscle sparing-none) includes the full width of the muscle; MS-1 includes preservation of the medial or lateral segment of the muscle; MS-2 includes the medial and lateral segment of the muscle; and the MS-3 includes preservation of all three segments. Free TRAM flaps are classified as MS-0, MS-1, and MS-2 (Fig. 4.11), whereas the DIEP flap is classified as MS-3 (Fig. 4.12).

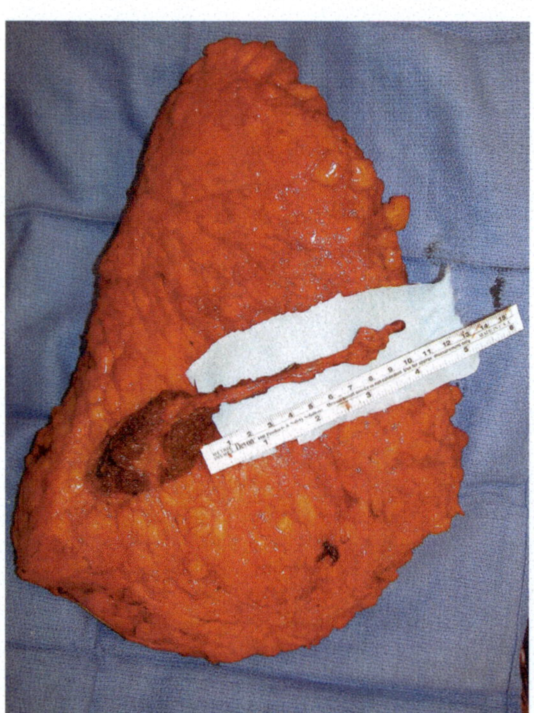

Fig. 4.11 A muscle-sparing free TRAM flap (MS-2) is shown

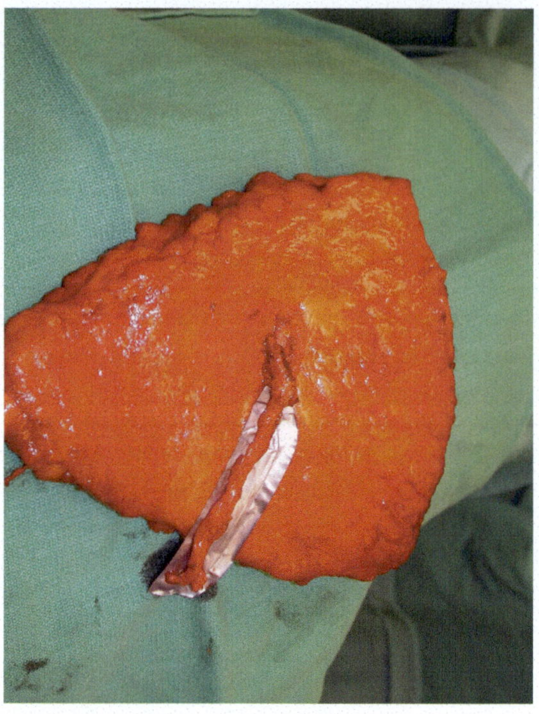

Fig. 4.12 A DIEP flap (MS-3) is shown

TRAM Flap

The pedicle TRAM flap utilizes the rectus abdominis muscle and is the only abdominal flap that does not require microvascular techniques [50]. The anatomy of the pedicle TRAM differs when compared to the other abdominal flaps. The primary vascularity is derived from the superior epigastric artery and vein. The primary purpose of the rectus abdominis muscle is that of a carrier for these vessels. It is not a significant source of breast volume except in women who are thin with small volume requirements. The advantages of the pedicle TRAM are that it is technically easier to perform, it can be performed without an assistant, and it does not require the use of an operating microscope or high-power loupes. Disadvantages of the pedicle TRAM are several-fold and related to perfusion capacity, because the superior epigastric artery and vein are usually less robust than the inferior epigastric artery and vein, abdominal weakness is due to greater muscle sacrifice, and contour abnormalities are due to loss of musculofacial support.

Free TRAM Flap

The free TRAM flap is similar to the pedicle TRAM flap in that it utilizes the same cutaneous territory of the abdomen [54]. The free TRAM requires microvascular surgery and therefore requires a recipient vessel that is usually the internal mammary or thoracodorsal artery and vein. The advantage of a free TRAM over a DIEP flap is that multiple perforators are included that may minimize the incidence of fat necrosis and venous congestion. Once a network of perforators is visualized; the anterior rectus sheath is outlined to encompass the perforators. The fascia is incised creating an island of perforators. It is important to preserve the lateral intercostal motor innervation to maintain function of the rectus abdominis muscle. The recipient vessels for the free TRAM include the internal mammary or the thoracodorsal artery and vein. Following flap harvest, the recipient vessels are anastomosed to the donor vessels using a suture technique or with a coupling device. Once the anastomosis is complete, the flap is inset and shaped to create a new breast mound. The abdominal closure includes reapproximation of the anterior rectus sheath with or without mesh support followed by layered skin closure. Figures 4.13 and 4.14 illustrate a patient following bilateral free TRAM reconstruction.

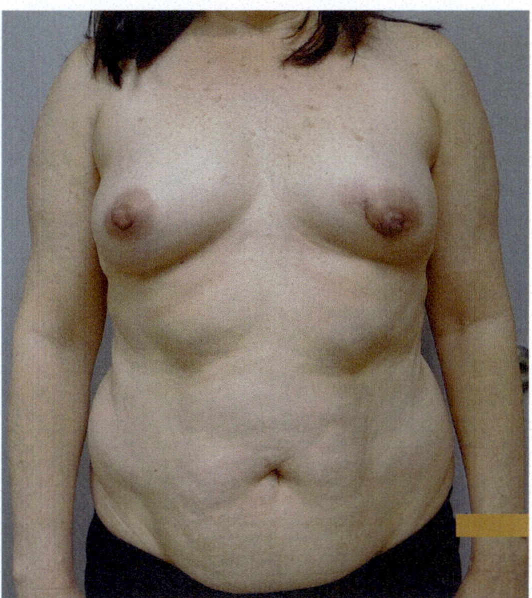

Fig. 4.13 Preoperative photograph of a woman with left breast cancer

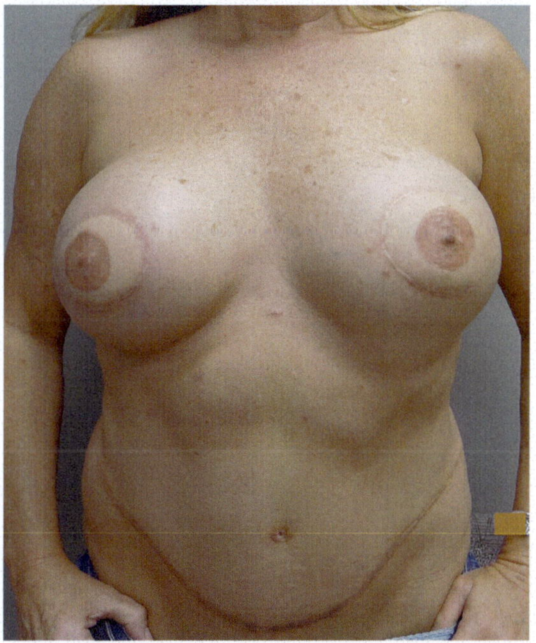

Fig. 4.14 Postoperative photography following bilateral skin-sparing mastectomy and bilateral MS-2 free TRAM flaps and delayed insertion of bilateral breast implants for volume enhancement

DIEP Flap

The DIEP flap is a true perforator flap as it isolates the primary source vessel of the flap and harvests it without removing any muscle [54]. A myotomy is necessary to dissect the deep inferior epigastric artery and vein. The decision regarding whether to perform an MS-2 free TRAM or DIEP flap is ultimately based on the presence and quality of the abdominal wall perforating vessels. Knowledge of these perforators can be assessed either pre- or intraoperatively. Preoperative assessment is best achieved using computed angiography (CT) or magnetic resonance (MR) angiography. With these techniques, the location and caliber of the perforating vessels can be adequately determined. If a dominant perforator arising from the deep system is not identified, it may be because the superficial inferior epigastric system is the more dominant. In this situation, one can consider performing an SIEA. During DIEP flap dissection, it is imperative to preserve the lateral intercostal nerves to preserve the motor function of the rectus abdominis muscle. Following the elevation and microvascular anastomosis, the flap is inset and the abdomen is closed (Figs. 4.15, 4.16, and 4.17).

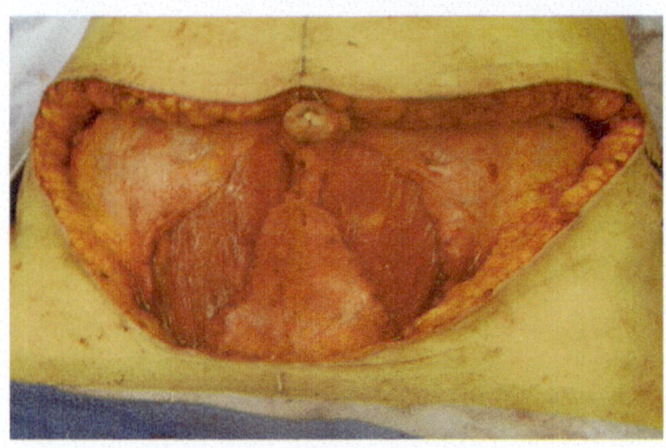

Fig. 4.16 Intraoperative photograph demonstrating complete preservation of the rectus abdominis muscle following bilateral DIEP flaps

SIEA Flap

The SIEA flap is an alternative abdominal flap option that is suitable in some women [62]. The SIEA flap is based on the superficial inferior epigastric artery and vein. The advantage of this flap over the other abdominal free flaps is that it does not require a fasciotomy or myotomy, thus the integrity of the abdominal wall is not disrupted. The superficial inferior epigastric vessels have been demonstrated to be "useable" in 30% of cases. The SIEA flap is technically easier to harvest than either the DIEP or muscle-sparing free TRAM flap because it is essentially an adipocutaneous flap that is perfused by a direct perforator. Direct perforators do not course through a muscle. A limitation of the SIEA flap is that the angiosome is usually confined to the ipsilateral flap; therefore, inclusion of zone 3 may result in inadequate perfusion and ultimately fat or partial flap necrosis. Thus, the SIEA flap is ideal for women having unilateral or bilateral breast reconstruction in which only a hemi flap is used.

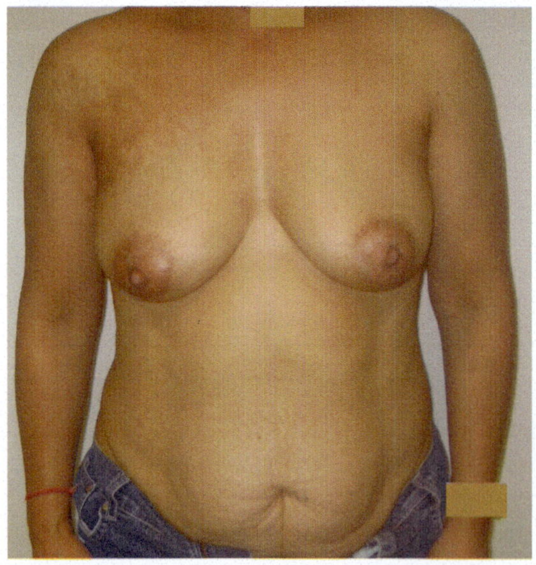

Fig. 4.15 Preoperative photograph of a woman with right breast cancer

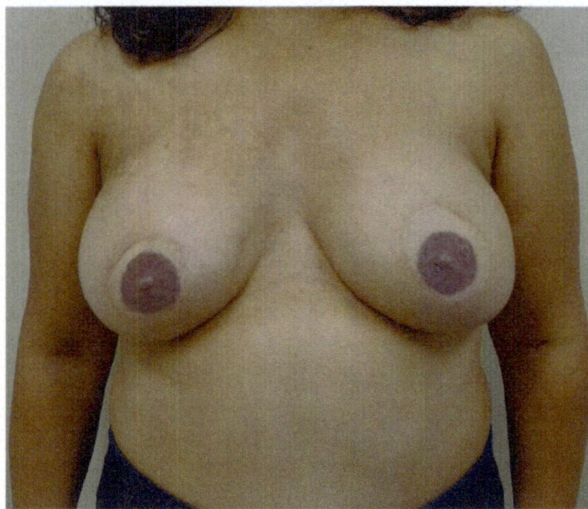

Fig. 4.17 Postoperative photography following bilateral skin-sparing mastectomy and bilateral DIEP flaps

Shaping the Abdominal Flap

There are several shaping advantages using free flaps for breast reconstruction. The flap is not tethered to the donor site muscle that allows for optimal positioning on the chest wall. The internal mammary vessels are the preferred recipient vessels and exposed at the level of the third or fourth costal rib segment. Alternatively, the thoracodorsal vessels can be used and are exposed in the axillary region. Because the thoracodorsal vessels are laterally based, bilateral reconstructions may sometimes result in a slight medial/sternal volume deficiency. This is usually not a problem with unilateral cases because zone 3 can supplement the medial breast.

When bilateral reconstruction with abdominal flaps is performed, the abdominal donor tissue is bisected at the midline such that each flap contains a zone 1 and zone 2. There are various positioning options for the flap on the chest wall that include placing the medial edge of the flap along the sternal border or along the inframammary fold. Suturing of the flap to the chest wall is sometimes necessary with immediate reconstruction especially when the footprint of the natural breast is larger than the footprint of the flap. These sutures can be placed superomedially, inferomedially, and laterally. With delayed reconstruction, the dimensions of the created subcutaneous pocket are made to match that of the flap.

When unilateral reconstruction with an abdominal flap is performed, it is important to achieve symmetry with the opposite breast. Assessment of patient expectations is critical to know if the opposite breast will be reduced, augmented, or left as is. The opposite breast is used as a template for the reconstruction. Typically, with a unilateral reconstruction, zones 1–3 and sometimes zone 4 are utilized depending on the amount of tissue required and the perfusion of the distal flap zones. Because there is usually more tissue with a unilateral flap (zones 1–3) compared to the bilateral flap (zones 1–2), there are more shaping options. The flap can be folded in a conical fashion or it can be folded laterally such that apical portion (zone 2) of the flap is tucked under zone 1 with zone 3 of the flap being positioned along the sternal border. With both maneuvers, the goal is to provide better projection. Suturing the flap laterally is always necessary and suturing the flap along the medial border is sometimes necessary.

Flap Insetting

When insetting the flap following a unilateral or bilateral reconstruction, it is recommended to sit the patient upright to approximately 45° to assess the position, symmetry, contour, and projection of the breast. In cases of a skin-sparing mastectomy, the skin territory to be exteriorized is delineated and the remainder of the flap is de-epithelized. When a nipple-sparing mastectomy has been performed, a Doppler is used to identify an arteriovenous signal and delineated with a 2-cm circle. With nipple-sparing mastectomy, the entire flap can be de-epithelized and buried or a small skin island can be exteriorized. In either case, an arteriovenous Doppler signal must be identified for monitoring. With free flaps, the vascular pedicle must be inspected to ensure that it is not twisted or kinked. With pedicle flaps, the tunneling of the flap can sometimes compress the muscle and blood supply; therefore, it is imperative to reassess the perfusion of the flap to ensure that the perfusion is intact. With delayed reconstruction, the lower mastectomy skin is usually excised and the inferior edge of the autologous flap is used to recreate the inframammary fold. With both skin-sparing and nipple-sparing mastectomy, the flap can be monitored using traditional monitoring techniques that include hand-held Doppler, assessment of capillary perfusion, and skin turgor.

Latissimus Dorsi Reconstruction

The latissimus dorsi musculocutaneous flap and the thoracodorsal artery perforator flap are two additional options for total or partial breast reconstruction [51, 57, 61]. These flaps are usually raised as pedicle flaps and do not require microvascular surgery. The thoracodorsal artery and vein constitute the primary blood supply for these flaps. Latissimus dorsi flaps are useful for immediate or delayed breast reconstruction. Disadvantages of the latissimus flap include donor site scarring, creation of asymmetry, and the frequent need for an implant and/or tissue expander. Autologous fat grating can be considered to augment volume, improve contour, and improve skin quality. The most common complication is seroma formation that occurs in approximately 5–25% of patients at the site of muscle harvest.

As with all reconstructions, the volume and skin requirements of the new breast are assessed and juxtaposed in relation to the estimated volume of the latissimus dorsi musculocutaneous flap. Because this flap provides a limited quantity of skin and fat, the use of a prosthetic device is sometimes required. In making this decision, it is important to assess the footprint, conus, and skin envelope on the natural breast. In the case of a volume deficiency, a tissue expander or permanent implant can be considered. This will also help to augment the projection of the breast in order to better define the desired conus. Other methods to obtain additional volume using the LD flap include beveling the fat away from the skin paddle in order to increase the quantity of fat harvested from the back [57]. Some surgeons' prefer to leave the thoracodorsal nerve intact to prevent muscle atrophy and to maintain greater volume. Others prefer to divide the nerve in order to prevent any animation that may occur with a contracting muscle. Figures 4.18, 4.19, 4.20, and 4.21 illustrate a patient who had a three-stage latissimus dorsi flap reconstruction.

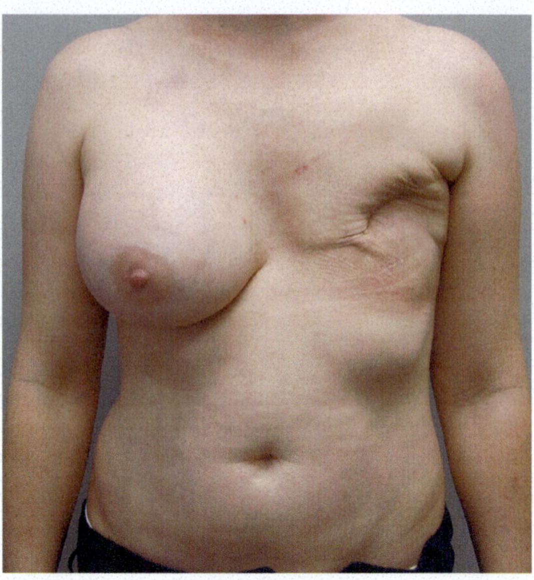

Fig. 4.18 Preoperative photograph of a woman following left skin-sparing mastectomy and radiation therapy

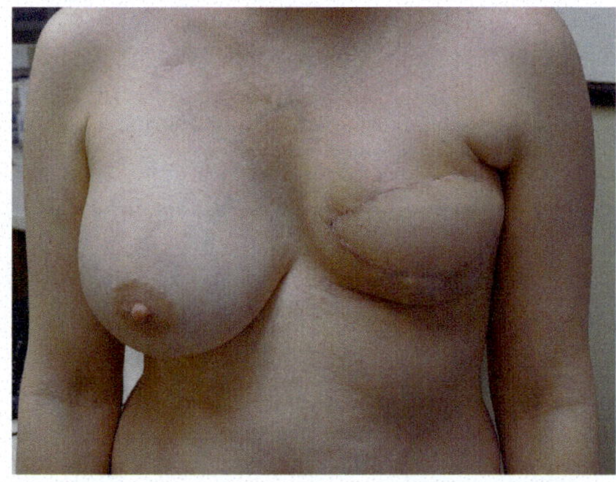

Fig. 4.19 Postoperative photograph following left breast reconstruction with the latissimus dorsi musculocutaneous flap

Gluteal Flaps

The gluteal flaps are arguably some of the more complex flaps in the armamentarium of the microsurgeon [53, 55, 60]. In general, these flaps

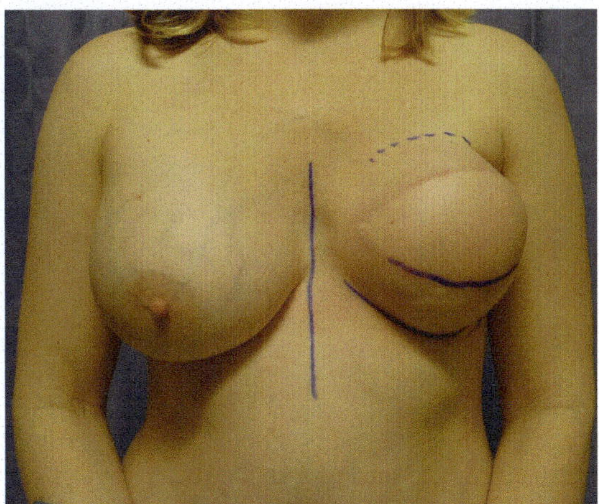

Fig. 4.20 Postoperative photograph following insertion of a tissue expander for volume enhancement demonstrating the preoperative marking for the exchange to a permanent implant

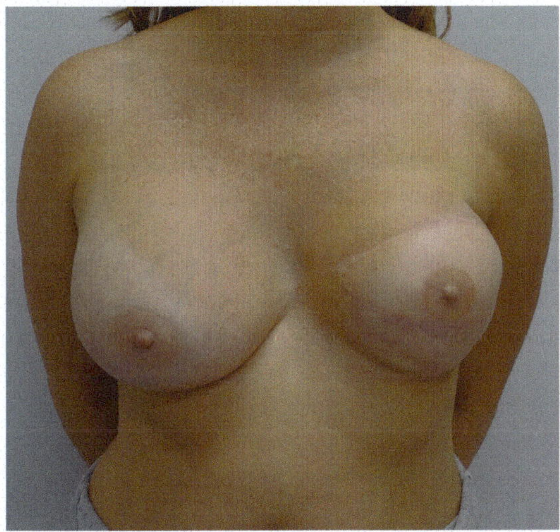

Fig. 4.21 Postoperative photograph demonstrating the latissimus dorsi flap with a permanent implant and nipple–areolar reconstruction

are considered when the abdomen is not a suitable donor site and the patient is not interested in prosthetic reconstruction. Gluteal flaps can be raised with or without the gluteus maximus muscle. There are two perforator flaps that are derived from this region that include the superior (SGAP) and inferior (IGAP) gluteal artery perforator flaps. The gluteal flaps are ideally suited for women who are of moderate body habitus and not usually recommended for obese women.

SGAP Flap

The technical aspects of harvesting gluteal flaps require special attention. Anatomic landmarks include the greater trochanter laterally, the posterior superior iliac crest superiorly, and the coccyx inferiorly. The location of the perforators is best determined using a hand-held Doppler probe with the patient in the prone position on the operating table. In contrast to the DIEP flap where a centrally based perforator is preferred, with the SGAP, a peripheral perforator is preferred to facilitate the microsurgical anastomosis and flap insetting. The dissection continues deep to the gluteus maximus and medius muscle before penetrating the deep fibrous fascia. Once the dissection is complete, the flap is harvested, the microvascular anastomosis is completed, and the flap is inset. Figures 4.22, 4.23, 4.24, and 4.25 illustrate a patient following bilateral SGAP flap reconstruction.

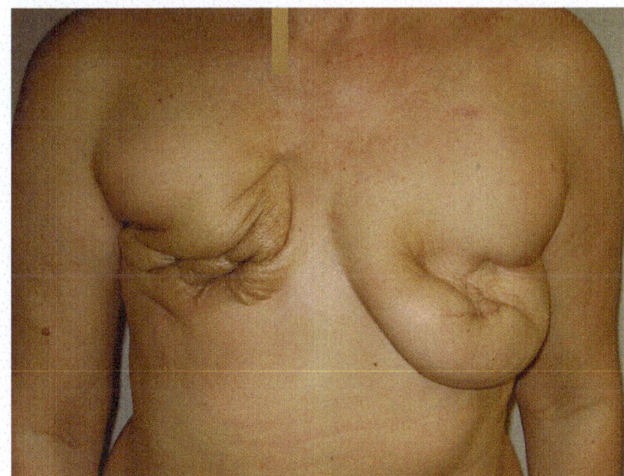

Fig. 4.22 Preoperative photograph of a woman following bilateral skin-sparing mastectomy, bilateral radiation therapy, and failed implant reconstruction

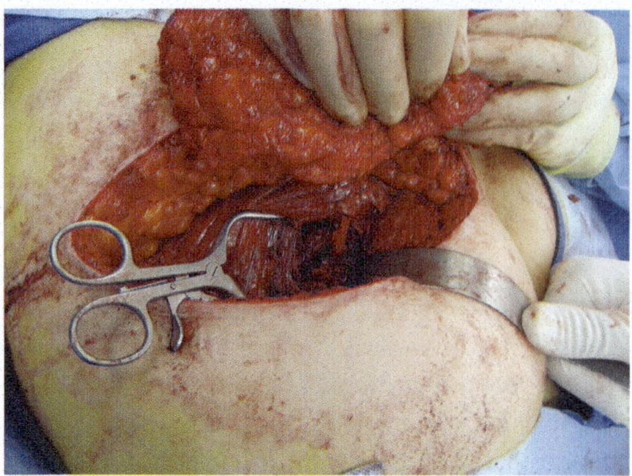

Fig. 4.23 Intraoperative photograph demonstrating the harvest of a SGAP flap

IGAP Flap

The IGAP flap is raised with the same landmarks as the SGAP flap; however, the skin territory for this flap is positioned along the inferior gluteal crease. In general, the adipocutaneous component of this flap is slightly less than that of the SGAP. Limitations of the IGAP flap are that the sciatic nerve is often exposed during this dissection and may result in postoperative discomfort. Because the incision is located in the ischial region, sitting may be restricted for several days following the operation and dehiscence of the incision may be observed more often.

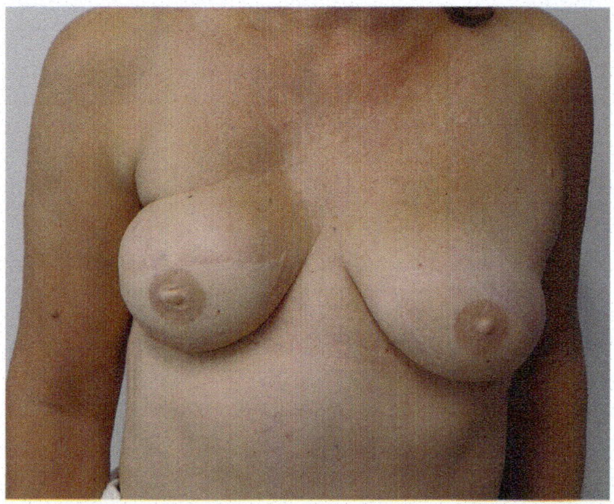

Fig. 4.24 Postoperative photograph following staged bilateral SGAP breast reconstruction and nipple–areolar reconstruction

Shaping Gluteal Flaps

Gluteal flaps tend to have a shorter vascular pedicle than the abdominal flaps and optimal positioning on the chest wall may be compromised. The dimensions of these flaps range from 12 to 25 cm in length to 6–10 cm in width and the thickness ranges from 4 to 8 cm. Shaping the SGAP flap is limited due to the thickness of the flap. However, designing the flap with a lateral extension can allow for a conical shaping to more naturally mimic the natural breast [72]. Secondary contouring of these flaps is sometimes necessary. In cases of delayed reconstruction where a gluteal flap is considered, pre-expansion of the breast skin to provide an increased skin envelope can improve aesthetic outcome [73].

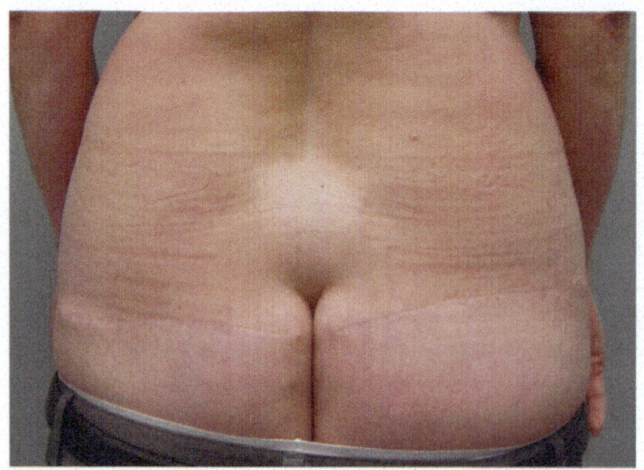

Fig. 4.25 Postoperative photograph demonstrating the appearance of the buttock donor site

Thigh Flaps

The medial and posterior thigh regions have become an excellent alternative donor site for autologous breast reconstruction. Flaps such as the transverse upper gracilis (TUG), transverse musculocutaneous gracilis (TMG), and the profunda artery perforator (PAP) have been utilized.

TUG and TMG Flaps

Candidates for a medially based thigh flap (TMG and TUG) include women with minimal abdominal fat or significant disruption of vascularity due to prior scars [52, 59, 63]. Candidates must have an excess of skin and fat in the medial thigh region. Other indications include bilateral reconstructions in which the mastectomy volume approximates the volume of the medial thigh or meets the expectation of the patient. Patients are evaluated in the standing position by pinching the medial thigh region to determine the optimal height of the flap. The skin paddle can be delineated transversely or in a Fleur-de-lis pattern. During the dissection, the gracilis muscle is visualized and divided at its origin and at its distal musculotendinous insertion. The flap is transferred to the chest wall for the microvascular anastomosis.

Shaping the breast using medial thigh flaps has been described [74]. The segment of gracillis muscle is usually placed along the area where the cartilaginous rib harvest has occurred to minimize visibility of this. Because of the added length of these flaps, they lend themselves nicely to coning by suturing the anterior and posterior edge of the flap together. The coned flap is positioned on the chest wall to ensure adequate coverage of the footprint and to generate adequate projection.

PAP Flap

The PAP flap is becoming the preferred second option for many surgeons [56]. This flap is based off the profunda femoris artery and vein that has several associated perforators within the posterior compartment of the thigh. This flap is often considered as an alternative to the abdomen and ideally suited for small-to-moderate size breasts with lipodystrophy in the posterior thigh territory. The weight of this flap ranges from 250 to 700 grams. The advantages of this flap over gluteal flaps and medial thigh flaps are that lymphedema risk is minimal, pedicle length is increased, and gluteal contour is not affected. The PAP flap can be easily shaped into a cone to provide optimal projection. The posterior thigh tissues are more pliable than the gluteal tissue and sometimes more pliable than the abdominal tissue that facilitates coning and achieving ideal aesthetics. Flap weight typically ranges from 250 to 600 grams and can be used unilaterally and bilaterally. The incidence of fat necrosis has been generally less than 10%. Secondary recontouring is usually not necessary.

Secondary Revisions

Secondary revisions are often necessary following autologous reconstruction [75]. This may be to restore volume, contour, and position. This may include both breasts in the setting of a bilateral reconstruction as well as the ipsilateral and contralateral breast in the setting of a unilateral reconstruction. Various techniques are available for the reconstructed breast that includes soft tissue recontouring, fat grafting, burying the flap, and implant placement. Achieving symmetry with a non-reconstructed breast can be achieved by augmentation, mastopexy, and reduction mammaplasty. Resorbable mesh products have demonstrated success in the setting of recurrent breast ptosis [76].

The Reconstructed Breast

Perhaps the most common method of revision is to recontour the soft tissue by direct excision of skin and fat as well as tissue rearrangement [75]. This can be performed to reduce the volume, improve the shape, reposition the breast on the chest wall, and to better define the inframammary or lateral mammary folds. The use of autologous fat grafting to correct contour deformities and to improve skin quality has become another common method of revision that has achieved success. The placement of fat along the upper pole of the breast and chest wall is an ideal method to achieve natural contours. Fat grafting has also been used in radiated breasts where skin damage is present. The ability of fat and stem cells to regenerate, hydrate, and improve the vascularity of the damaged skin has been described [36]. For the autologous reconstruction that remains too ptotic, the technique of burying the flap has demonstrated success. The skin territory is outlined with an elliptical extension and de-epithelized. The mastectomy skin flaps are undermined superiorly and inferiorly and then reapproximated.

For the reconstructed breast that is deficient in volume, two methods of correction are commonly employed. The first is to fat graft the substance of the flap and the second is to place a small implant under the flap. The implant can be saline or silicone and ranges in volume from 80 to 125 cc. In women with a history of chest wall radiation, the device is placed in the prepectoral position, whereas in women without a history of radiation therapy, the device is usually placed in the subpectoral position.

The Non-reconstructed Breast

In unilateral reconstructions, the non-reconstructed breast is sometimes modified to achieve symmetry [77]. Options include unilateral augmentation with an implant, mastopexy, and reduction mammaplasty. Implant selection is facilitated by volumetric analysis using three-dimensional imaging. The technique is essentially that of a standard breast augmentation. When volumes are similar but the natural breast is ptotic, a mastopexy is often performed. This is usually via a circumvertical approach; however, when extreme, inverted T techniques are performed. When the reconstructed breast is smaller than the natural breast, reduction mammaplasty is usually performed. This can be performed using a variety of techniques that include short scars when the difference is mild to moderate and inverted T scars when the difference is moderate to severe.

Conclusion

Breast reconstruction following mastectomy continues to evolve with the goal of improving surgical and aesthetic outcomes. The ability to successfully reconstruct a breast with prosthetic devices or autologous tissues has become predictable and reproducible based on proper patient selection, attention to detail, and modern technical approaches related to the mastectomy and the reconstruction.

Disclosure Dr. Nahabedian is a consultant for Allergan and Chief Surgical Officer at PolarityTE.

Editorial Comments This important chapter addresses the reconstructive options for breast cancer patients and describes the necessary considerations needed in shaping an aesthetically appealing breast. Dr. Nahabedian's practice has certainly given him the opportunity to be a pioneer in this field with vast experience in both alloplastic reconstruction and autologous reconstruction.

Dr. Nahabedian does an excellent job of describing not only the surgical techniques but also the importance of patient selection; timing of the surgery, be it immediate or delayed immediate; and choice of the right operation for the right patient. One useful tool that I use in my practice to decide between immediate or delayed immediate reconstruction is the breast risk assessment (BRA) score calculator. It takes into account patients' comorbidities and provides a percentage for their risk profile. In general, I delay any patient with BRA score higher than 20% in order to reduce their perioperative risks. In addition, by sharing this number with the patient, she has a better understanding of the reason for the delay.

Dr. Nahabedian also highlights the importance of muscle preservation in both the prepectoral implant-based and perforator flap breast reconstructions, when feasible. I, however, want to emphasize that this decision must be made in consultation with the patient's oncological team to ensure concordance in proper monitoring as it pertains to postoperative surveillance for local recurrence.

Dr. Nahabedian lists some of the presumed indications for the use of ADM in prepectoral and subpectoral alloplastic reconstruction. At the time of this writing, there are also some emerging data that show that partial pocket reinforcement with mesh scaffold can provide pocket stability laterally or inferiorly and we can achieve as good a result as with full or partial coverage of prosthesis with ADM without seeing a rise in some of the feared complications of prepectoral reconstruction, i.e., capsular contracture. However, Dr. Nahabedian rightfully states about ADM: "Although used by many plastic surgeons, controversy regarding its use remains." In fact, at the time of this writing, the use of ADM and mesh scaffold in breast surgery is considered off-label by FDA due to lack of prospective head-to-head data to establish the efficacy of these products in breast reconstruction.

Dr. Nahabedian also highlights the challenges in reconstructing patients with breast hypertrophy. He describes the three features that influence breast shape as being the footprint, conus, and skin envelope. He states that most women in this category have excess skin and require skin reduction. He states that the two common mastectomy incisions in these patients include the inverted T incision and the extended transverse/oblique skin excision pattern. I use a variation of transverse incision that I call the smile-pattern skin excision. This provides both transverse and vertical skin reduction while preserving a dermal flap, which, by advancing it under the superior skin flap, provides extra thickness to the upper pole. In addition, the nipple–areola complex graft can be either included as part of the dermal flap or added as garft onto the upper skin flap. Furthermore, in unilateral cases when performing contralateral reduction or mastopexy, the symmetry of the lower pole can be improved by using a mesh scaffold as an internal sling to support and stabilize the lower pole tissue (see case study in Chap. 5).

Congratulations again to Dr. Nahabedian on his excellent chapter and pioneering work in shaping the breast in reconstruction.

Kiya Movassaghi

References

1. Maxwell GP, Gabriel A. Bioengineered breast: concept, technique, and preliminary results. Plast Reconstr Surg. 2016;137(2):415–21.
2. American Society of Plastic Surgeons Procedural Statistics. www.plasticsurgery.org. Accessed 11 Oct 2018.
3. Albornoz CR, Bach PB, Mehrara BJ, Disa JJ, Pusic AL, McCarthy CM, et al. A paradigm shift in U.S. breast reconstruction: increasing implant rates. Plast Reconstr Surg. 2013;131:15.
4. Cemal Y, Albornoz CR, Disa JJ, McCarthy CM, Mehrara BJ, Pusic AL, et al. A paradigm shift in U.S. breast reconstruction: part 2. The influence of changing mastectomy patterns on reconstructive rate and method. Plast Reconstr Surg. 2013;131:320e.
5. McCarthy CM, Mehrara BJ, Riedel E, Davidge K, Hinson A, Disa JJ, et al. Predicting complications following expander/implant breast reconstruction: an outcomes analysis based on preoperative clinical risk. Plast Reconstr Surg. 2008;121:1886.
6. Nahabedian MY. Current approaches to prepectoral breast reconstruction. Plast Reconstr Surg. 2018;142(4):871–80.
7. Rebowe RE, Allred L, Nahabedian MY. The evolution from subcutaneous to prepectoral prosthetic breast reconstruction. Plast Reconstr Surg Glob Open. 2018;6(6):e1797.
8. Nahabedian MY. Breast reconstruction: a review and rationale for patient selection. Plast Reconstr Surg. 2009;124:55–62.
9. Dietz J, Lundgren P, Veeramani A, O'Rourke C, Bernard S, Djohan R, et al. Autologous inferior dermal sling (autoderm) with concomitant skin-envelope reduction mastectomy: an excellent surgical choice for women with macromastia and clinically significant ptosis. Ann Surg Oncol. 2012;19(10):3282–8.
10. Rinker B, Thornton BP. Skin-sparing mastectomy and immediate tissue expander breast reconstruction in patients with macromastia using the Passot breast reduction pattern. Ann Plast Surg. 2014;72(6):S158–64.
11. Rammos CK, Mammolito D, King VA, Yoo A. Two-stage reconstruction of the large and ptotic breasts: skin reduction mastectomy with prepectoral device placement. Plast Reconstr Surg Glob Open. 2018;6(7):e1853.
12. Antony AK, Mehrara BM, McCarthy CM, et al. Salvage of tissue expanders in the setting of mastectomy flap necrosis: 13 years experience using timed excision with continued expansion. Plast Reconstr Surg. 2009;124:356–263.
13. Patel KM, Hill LM, Gatti ME, Nahabedian MY. Management of massive mastectomy skin flap necrosis following autologous breast reconstruction. Ann Plast Surg. 2012;69:139–44.
14. Matsen CB, Mehrara B, Eaton A, Capko D, Berg A, Stempel M, et al. Skin flap necrosis after mastectomy with reconstruction: a prospective study. Ann Surg Oncol. 2016;23(1):257–64.
15. Yalanis GC, Naq S, Georgek JR, Cooney CM, Manahan MA, Rosson GD, et al. Mastectomy weight and tissue expander volume predict necrosis and increased costs associated with breast reconstruction. Plast Reconstr Surg Glob Open. 2015;3(7):e450.
16. Komorowska-Timek E, Gurtner G. Intraoperative perfusion mapping with laser-assisted indocyanine green imaging can predict and prevent complications in immediate breast reconstruction. Plast Reconstr Surg. 2010;125:1065–73.
17. Gdalevitch P, Van Lacken N, Bahng S, Ho A, Bovill E, Lennox P, et al. Effects of nitroglycerin ointment on mastectomy flap necrosis in immediate breast reconstruction: a randomized controlled trial. Plast Reconstr Surg. 2015;135(6):1530–9.
18. Zenn MR. Staged immediate breast reconstruction. Plast Reconstr Surg. 2015;135:976.
19. Paydar KZ, Wirth GA, Mowlds DS. Prepectoral breast reconstruction with fenestrated acellular dermal matrix: a novel design. Plast Reconstr Surg Glob Open. 2018;6(4):e1712.
20. Jones G, Yoo A, King V, Jao B, Wang H, Rammos C, et al. Prepectoral immediate direct-to-implant breast reconstruction with anterior AlloDerm coverage. Plast Reconstr Surg. 2017;140(6S Prepectoral Breast Reconstruction):31S–8S.
21. Kim JYS, Miodinow AS. What's new in acellular dermal matrix and soft-tissue support for prosthetic breast reconstruction. Plast Reconstr Surg. 2017;140(5S Advances in Breast Reconstruction):30S–43S.
22. Sbitany H, Serletti JM. Acellular dermis–assisted prosthetic breast reconstruction: a systematic and critical review of efficacy and associated morbidity. Plast Reconstr Surg. 2011;128:1162.
23. Kim JYS, Davila AA, Persing S. A meta-analysis of human acellular dermis and submuscular tissue expander breast reconstruction. Plast Reconstr Surg. 2012;129:28.
24. Salibian AA, Frey JD, Choi M, Karp NS. Subcutaneous implant-based breast reconstruction with acellular dermal matrix/mesh: a systematic review. Plast Reconstr Surg Glob Open. 2016;4(11):e1139.

25. Salzberg CA. Nonexpansive immediate breast reconstruction using human acellular tissue matrix graft (AlloDerm). Ann Plast Surg. 2006;57:1–5.
26. Nahabedian MY. Acellular dermal matrices in primary breast reconstruction: principles, concepts, and indications. Plast Reconstr Surg. 2012;130:5S–2. 44-53
27. Salzberg CA, Ashikari AY, Koch RM, Chabner-Thompson E. An 8-year experience of direct-to-implant immediate breast reconstruction using human acellular dermal matrix (AlloDerm). Plast Reconstr Surg. 2011;127:514.
28. Colwell AS, Damjanovic B, Zahedi B, Medford-Davis L, Hertl C, Austen WG Jr. Retrospective review of 331 consecutive immediate single-stage implant reconstructions with acellular dermal matrix: indications, complications, trends, and costs. Plast Reconstr Surg. 2011;128:1170.
29. Spear SL, Seruya M, Rao SS, Rottman S, Stolle E, Cohen M, et al. Two-stage prosthetic breast reconstruction using AlloDerm including outcomes of different timings of radiotherapy. Plast Reconstr Surg. 2012;130(1):1–9.
30. Nahabedian MY, Mesbahi AN. Breast reconstruction with tissue expanders and implants. In: Nahabedian MY, editor. Cosmetic and reconstructive breast surgery. London: Elsevier; 2009. p. 1–19.
31. Woo A, Harless C, Jacobsen SR. Revisiting an old place: single surgeon experience on post-mastectomy subcutaneous implant based breast reconstruction. Plast Reconstr Surg. 2015;136(4S-1(Supplement)):83.
32. Reitsamer R, Peintinger F. Prepectoral implant placement and complete coverage with porcine acellular dermal matrix: a new technique for direct-to-implant breast reconstruction after nipple-sparing mastectomy. J Plast Reconstr Aesth Surg. 2015;68:162–7.
33. Sigalove S. Options in acellular dermal matrix-device assembly. Plast Reconstr Surg. 2017;140(6S Prepectoral Breast Reconstruction):39S–42S.
34. Kaoutzanis C, Xin M, Ballard NS, et al. Outcomes of autologous fat grafting following breast reconstruction in post-mastectomy patients. Plast Reconstr Surg (Supplement). 2014;134:4S–1.
35. Seth AK, Hirsch EM, Kim JYS, Fine NA. Long-term outcomes following fat grafting in prosthetic breast reconstruction: a comparative analysis. Plast Reconstr Surg. 2012;130:984.
36. Rigotti G, Marchi A, Galie M, Baroni G, Benati D, Krampera M, et al. Clinical treatment of radiotherapy tissue damage by lipoaspirate transplant: a healing process mediated by adipose-derived adult stem cells. Plast Reconstr Surg. 2007;119:1409.
37. Wang CF, Zhou Z, Yan YJ, Zhao DM, Chen F, Qiao Q. Clinical analyses of clustered microcalcifications after autologous fat injection for breast augmentation. Plast Reconstr Surg. 2011;127:1669–73.
38. Mineda K, Kuno S, Kato H, Kinoshita K, Doi K, Hashimoto I, et al. Chronic inflammation and progressive calcification as a result of fat necrosis: the worst outcome in fat grafting. Plast Reconstr Surg. 2014;133:1064–72.
39. Smith P, Adams WP, Lipchitz AH, Chau B, Sorokin E, Rohrich RJ, et al. Autologous human fat grafting: effect of harvesting and preparation techniques on adipocyte graft survival. Plast Reconstr Surg. 2006;117:1836.
40. Choi M, Small K, Levovitz C, Lee C, Fadi A, Karp NS. The volumetric analysis of fat graft survival in breast reconstruction. Plast Reconstr Surg. 2013;131(2):185–91.
41. Khouri RK, Smit JM, Cardoso E, Pallua N, Lantieri L, Mathijssen IM, et al. Percutaneous aponeurectomy and lipofilling: a regenerative alternative to breast reconstruction. Plast Reconstr Surg. 2013;132:1280–90.
42. Kronowitz SJ, Robb GL. Radiation therapy and breast reconstruction: a critical review of the literature. Plast Reconstr Surg. 2009;124:395.
43. Nahabedian MY. The impact of breast reconstruction on the oncologic efficacy of radiation therapy: a retrospective analysis. Ann Plast Surg. 2008;60:244–50.
44. Nahabedian MY. AlloDerm performance in the setting of breast implants, infection, and radiation. Plast Reconstr Surg. 2009;124:1735–40.
45. Seruya M, Cohen M, Rao S, et al. Two-stage prosthetic breast reconstruction using AlloDerm: a 7-year experience in irradiated and nonirradiated breasts. Plast Reconstr Surg. 2011;125:22–3.
46. Sigalove S, Maxwell GP, Sigalove NM, Storm-Dickerson TL, Pope N, Rice J, et al. Prepectoral implant-based breast reconstruction and postmastectomy radiotherapy: short-term outcomes. Plast Reconstr Surg Glob Open. 2017;6:e1631.
47. Elswick SM, Harless CA, Bishop SN, Schleck CD, Mandrekar J, Reusche RD, et al. Prepectoral implant-based breast reconstruction with postmastectomy radiation therapy. Plast Reconstr Surg. 2018;142:1.
48. Cordeiro PG, Albornoz CR, McCormick B, Hudis CA, Hu Q, Heerdt A, et al. What is the optimum timing of postmastectomy radiotherapy in two-stage prosthetic reconstruction: radiation to the tissue expander or permanent implant? Plast Reconstr Surg. 2015;135:1509.
49. Nava MB, Pennati AE, Lozza L, Spano A, Zambetti M, Catanuto G. Outcome of different timings of radiotherapy in implant-based breast reconstructions. Plast Reconstr Surg. 2011;128:353.
50. Tan BK, Loethy J, Ong YS, Ho GH, Pribaz JJ. Preferred use of the ipsilateral pedicled TRAM flap for immediate breast reconstruction: an illustrated approach. Aesthet Plast Surg. 2012;36(1):128–33.
51. Zhi L, Mohan AT, Vijayasekaran A, Hou C, Sur YJ, Morse M, Saint-Cyr M. Maximizing the volume of latissimus dorsi flap in autologous breast reconstruction with simultaneous multisite fat grafting. Aesthet Surg J. 2016;36(2):169–78.
52. Vega SJ, Sandeen SN, Bossert RP, Perrone A, Ortiz L, Herrera H. Gracilis myocutaneous free flap in autologous breast reconstruction. Plast Reconstr Surg. 2009;124:1400–9.

53. Ahmadzadeh R, Bergeron L, Tang M, Morris S. The superior and inferior gluteal artery perforator flaps. Plast Reconstr Surg. 2007;120:1551–6.
54. Nahabedian MY, Momen B, Tsangaris T. Breast reconstruction with the muscle sparing (MS-2) free TRAM and the DIEP flap: is there a difference? Plast Reconstr Surg. 2005;115:436–44.
55. Allen RJ, Levine JL, Granzow JW. The in-the-crease inferior gluteal artery perforator flap for breast reconstruction. Plast Reconstr Surg. 2006;118:333–9.
56. Allen RJ, Haddock NT, Ahn CY, Sadeghi A. Breast reconstruction with the profunda artery perforator flap. Plast Reconstr Surg. 2012;129:16e.
57. Angrigiani C, Rancati A, Escudero E, Artero G. Extended thoracodorsal artery perforator flap for breast reconstruction. Gland Surg. 2015;4(6):519–27.
58. Chevray PM. Brest reconstruction with superficial inferior epigastric artery flaps: a prospective comparison with TRAM and DIEP flaps. Plast Reconstr Surg. 2004;114:1077–83.
59. Dayan E, Smith ML, Sultan M, Samson W, Dayan JH. The diagonal upper gracilis (DUG) flap: a safe and improved alternative to the TUG flap. Plast Reconstr Surg. 2013;132(4s-1):33–34.
60. Guerra AB, Metzinger SE, Bidros RS, Gill PS, Dupin CA, Allen RJ. Breast reconstruction with gluteal artery perforator flaps: a critical analysis of 142 flaps. Ann Plast Surg. 2004;52:118–24.
61. Heitmann C, Guerra A, Metzinger SW, Levin LS, Allen RJ. The thoracodorsal artery perforator flap: anatomic basis and clinical applications. Ann Plast Surg. 2003;51:23–9.
62. Holm C, Mayr M, Hofter E, Ninkivic M. The versatility of the SIEA flap: a clinical assessment of the vascular territory of the superficial epigastric inferior artery. J Plast Reconstr Aesthet Surg. 2007;60: 946–51.
63. Schoeller T, Huemer GM, Wechselberger G. The transverse musculocutaneous gracillis flap for breast reconstruction: guidelines for flap and patient selection. Plast Reconstr Surg. 2008;122:29–38.
64. Blondeel PN, Hijawi J, Depypere H, Roche N, Van Landuyt K. Shaping the breast in aesthetic and reconstructive breast surgery: an easy three- step principle. Plast Reconstr Surg. 2009;123:455.
65. Blondeel PN, Hijawi J, Depypere H, Roche N, Van Landuyt K. Shaping the breast in aesthetic and reconstructive breast surgery: an easy three-step principle. Part II—breast reconstruction after total mastectomy. Plast Reconstr Surg. 2009;123:794.
66. Blondeel PN, Hijawi J, Depypere H, Roche N, Van Landuyt K. Shaping the breast in aesthetic and reconstructive breast surgery: an easy three-step principle. Part III—reconstruction following breast conservative treatment. Plast Reconstr Surg. 2009; 124:28.
67. Blondeel PN, Hijawi J, Depypere H, Roche N, Van Landuyt K. Shaping the breast in aesthetic and reconstructive breast surgery: an easy three-step principle. Part IV—aesthetic breast surgery. Plast Reconstr Surg. 2009;124:372.
68. Mallucci P, Branford OA. Population analysis of the perfect breast: a morphometric analysis. Plast Reconstr Surg. 2014;134:436.
69. Nahabedian MY. Secondary operations of the anterior abdominal wall following microvascular breast reconstruction with the TRAM and DIEP flaps. Plast Reconstr Surg. 2007;120:365–72.
70. Nahabedian MY, Dooley W, Singh N, Manson PN. Contour abnormalities of the abdomen following breast reconstruction with abdominal flaps: the role of muscle preservation. Plast Reconstr Surg. 2002;109:91–101.
71. Nahabedian MY, Manson PN. Contour abnormalities of the abdomen following TRAM flap breast reconstruction: a multifactorial analysis. Plast Reconstr Surg. 2002;109:81–7.
72. Kronowicz SJ. Redesigned gluteal artery perforator flap for breast reconstruction. Plast Reconstr Surg. 2008;121:728.
73. Gurunluoglu R, Spanio S, Rainer C, Ninkovic M. Skin expansion before breast reconstruction with the superior gluteal artery perforator flap improves aesthetic outcome. Ann Plast Surg. 2003;50:475–9.
74. Fansa H, Schimer S, Warnecke IC, Cervelli A, Frerichs O. The transverse myocutaneous gracilis muscle flap: a fast and reliable method for breast reconstruction. Plast Reconstr Surg. 2008;122(5):1326–33.
75. Nahabedian MY. Symmetrical breast reconstruction: analysis of secondary procedures following reconstruction with implants and with autologous tissue. Plast Reconstr Surg. 2005;115:257–60.
76. Adams WP, Moses AC. Use of poly-4-hydroxybutyrate mesh to optimize soft-tissue support in mastopexy: a single-site study. Plast Reconstr Surg. 2017;139(1):67–75.
77. Nahabedian MY. Managing the opposite breast: contralateral symmetry procedures. Cancer J. 2008;14:258–63.

5 Shaping the Breast: Managing Complex Breast Issues

Kiya Movassaghi and Kevin J. Shultz

Introduction

Implant breast surgery continues to be one of the most frequently performed surgeries by plastic surgeons; yet, it has one of the highest numbers of revisionary surgeries, which can be as high as 30–40% [1–3]. The most common reasons for revision surgery include capsular contracture, implant malposition, asymmetry, implant rupture, desire for size change, ptosis, wrinkling/rippling, or hematoma/seroma [3, 4]. There are also challenging cases such as tuberous breast, aging or atrophied breast tissues, breast asymmetry, and certain chest wall anatomies that require a thoughtful and methodical approach in order to have a successful outcome. The three determinants of successful implant-based breast surgery (patient factors, implant factors, and surgical factors) have been discussed thoroughly in Chap. 1. Adhering to these guiding principles will help the surgeon achieve a more predictable outcome with improved patient satisfaction. However, even the most adept surgeons will still face these challenges. The purpose of this chapter is to discuss the management of some of these complex issues through a series of case presentations.

The Constricted Lower Pole

The constricted lower pole, meaning a short N-IMF distance and a tight tissue envelope, is challenging to deal with. If not handled correctly, the implant may sit higher on the chest with a less than ideal ratio of width to lower pole (see Chap. 1). In addition, patient's existing breast tissue and skin can end up as a visible mass on top of the lower middle part of the implants, causing a so-called double bubble. This happens due to persistence of tissue memory that occurs if the native inferior circummammary ligament (IMF) has been preserved. In order to avoid these, the surgeon should (1) lower the IMF according to the implant base width and implant surface being used (see the algorithms for lowering the IMF for smooth and textured implants in Chap. 1); (2) score the IMF and tight bands from underneath (radial release); (3) create dual-plane II pocket if performing subpectoral augmentation to allow for more implant–parenchyma exposure; (4) use implants containing highly cohesive gel; and (5) consider subfascial augmentation, which eliminates the influence of the pectoralis muscle and lowers the risk of double-bubble deformity (our preference). In many of these cases, periareolar mastopexy is also necessary to reduce the nipple areolar complex projec-

K. Movassaghi (✉)
Clinical Assistant Professor of Plastic Surgery, Oregon Health & Science University, Portland, OR, USA

Movassaghi Plastic Surgery & Ziba Medical Spa, Eugene, OR, USA

ASAPS Endorsed Aesthetic Fellowship, Eugene, OR, USA
e-mail: kiya@drmovassaghi.com

K. J. Shultz
Upstate Plastic Surgery, Greer, SC, USA

K. Movassaghi (ed.), *Shaping the Breast*, https://doi.org/10.1007/978-3-030-59777-1_5

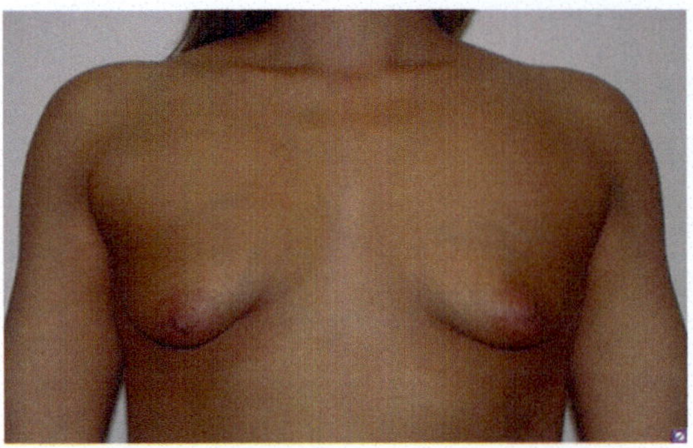

Fig. 5.1

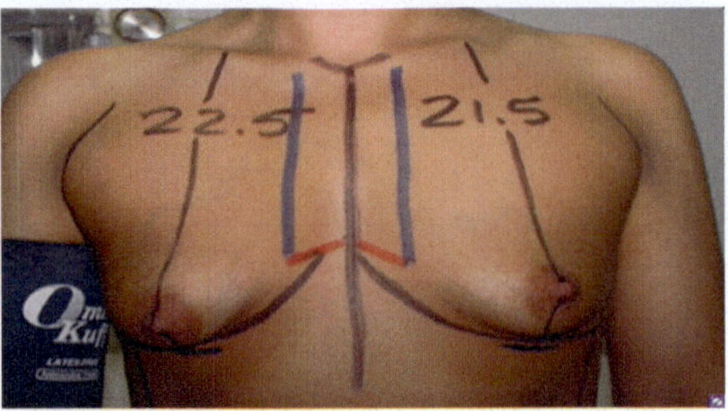

Fig. 5.2

tion, which gives the appearance of a wider breast. Highly cohesive implants (smooth and textured) working as controlled tissue expanders in a precise pocket with juxtaposition of breast parenchyma and implant will modulate the tissue positively in a period of many months postoperatively, expanding the lower pole tissue in an anterocaudal direction, depending on the shape of implant (a stronger action–reaction, Newton's third law). This forces the tissue to drape the implant nicely. Scoring of the breast tissue releases tight strands of connective tissue (Superficial Fascia System (SFS) and IMF tissues), enabling the tissue to spread out over the anterior and lower surface of the implant and help reduce the "memory" of native IMF tissues.

Case Analysis

A 30-year-old female presented with postpartum atrophy in the setting of tuberous breast with asymmetry. On examination, she had ptotic breasts (grade 2 on the left and grade 3 on the right) with constricted bases and short N-IMF distances in the setting of a high footprint and a very convex upper chest (Fig. 5.1). After discussing her options, she chose tear-shaped implants in the submuscular pocket to minimize upper pole fullness and visibility with her preexisting convexity.

She underwent bilateral dual-plane II augmentation with tear-shaped implants with lowering of IMF and radial release with periareolar mastopexy. Note that the IMF incision site and not her native IMF determined the new IMF (Fig. 5.2) (see our algorithm for lowering IMF for a textured implant in Chap. 1).

Postoperative photos at 1 year show good symmetry with controlled lower pole expansion and adequate upper pole fullness in light of her natural bony convexity (Fig. 5.3). Note that the location of new IMF coincides with the location of IMF incision site.

Also note that the controlled tissue expansion of the lower pole has continued postoperatively over the course of 12 months when compared to the 3 months postoperative exam without losing the stability at the IMF (Fig. 5.4).

Asymmetries

The source(s) of asymmetry can be multifactorial, and a precise diagnosis and treatment plan require a thorough examination of the trunk, including the ribcage and breasts. There is a strong correlation between asymmetries of breasts and chest wall deformities. Features such as scoliosis, ribcage profile (concave or convex), spinal rotation, and sternal contour (pectus excavatum, pectus carinatum) can greatly influence the breast shape and, hence, symmetry. In addition, inherent breast shape or volume asymmetries can be the underlying cause. It is of paramount importance to note these features and bring them to the patient's attention, because they will influence the final outcome and symmetry. Patients must be reminded that not all these asymmetries are correctable and, at times, improvement is the best we can achieve. The surgeon may need to consider all his/her options, such as using different implant dimensions (*X*, *Y*, and *Z*), volume adjustments with excision or

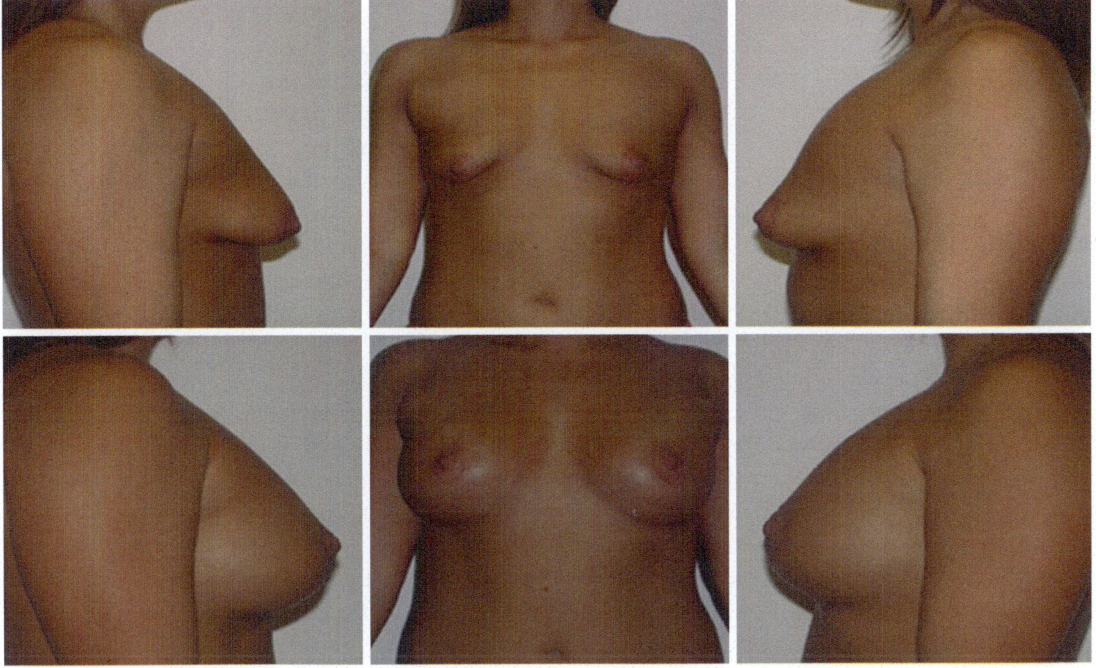

Fig. 5.3

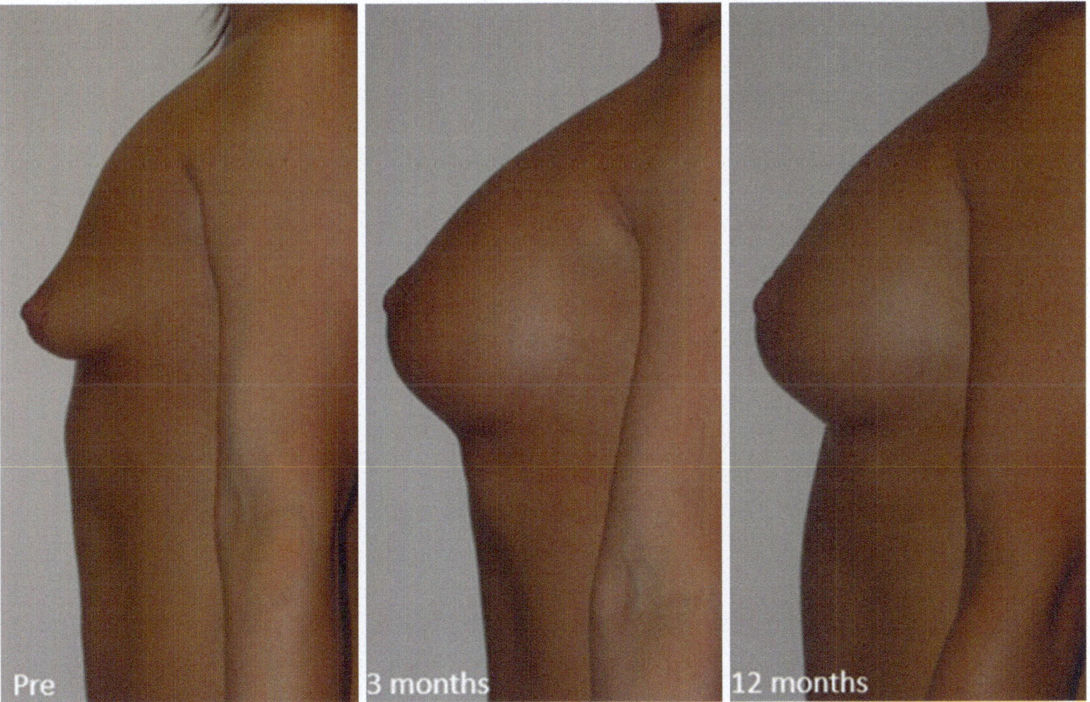

Fig. 5.4

liposuction, fat injection and differential skin envelope adjustments, and use of mesh to address some of these challenging issues.

Case Analysis

A 27-year-old female with no previous pregnancy presented for improved proportionality after undergoing a 40-pound weight loss that resulted in breast atrophy (Fig. 5.5). Her examination revealed a larger right breast but with more upper pole convexity on the left side, a relatively wide breast with short vertical height and upper chest. The breasts had different shapes, with the right side having a more constricted base and the left side having a more rounded base. She had grade 2 ptosis on the right side and grade 1 ptosis on the left side. The right IMF is higher than the left side by 0.5 cm. The left nipple is higher than the right by 1 cm. She has a scoliosis, with the left shoulder being higher.

After trying on sizers, she chose tear-shaped implants over the round ones due to her short upper chest and her desire for more natural appearance. Given the asymmetry in the upper chest convexities and breast projections, we chose different volumes for both sides by only increasing the z dimension on the left side while keeping the x and y dimensions the same (right side 320 cc 12.5/11.6/4.6 vs. left side 335 cc 12.5/11.6/5.1).

She underwent bilateral submuscular augmentation with dual-plane II on the right (constricted base) and dual-plane I on the left side. The IMF incision site was made lower than the native ones based on the algorithm, and the right IMF was further lowered 0.5 cm to improve the vertical discrepancy between the two sides (Fig. 5.6). Radial releases were also made to encourage

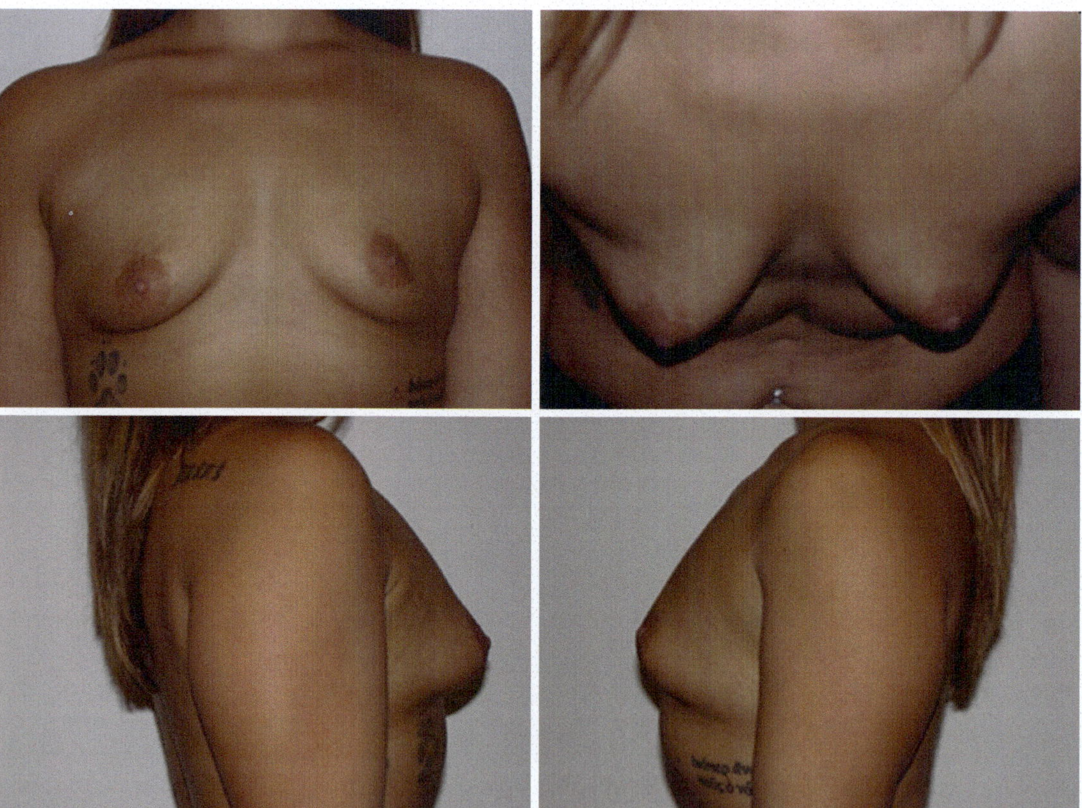

Fig. 5.5

further widening of the lower poles. Periareolar mastopexies were performed to make the nipple areolar complex (NACs) more symmetrical and make breast look more rounded.

Photos taken 14 months postoperatively show much improved symmetry in nipple location, shape, and projection, with good proportionality and pocket stability (Fig. 5.7).

Case Analysis

A 21-year-old G0 female presented for correction of breast asymmetry, more volume in the upper pole, and a lift (Fig. 5.8). She developed significant asymmetry after puberty. She liked the volume of the left breast in a bra with more fullness in the upper pole. Her examination revealed bilateral grade 3 ptosis with the left breast larger than the right in the setting of low footprint. In addition, she had lipodystrophy of her axillary folds and tails.

Treatment-wise, she had two options. She could choose to have augmentation and mastopexy on the right side and mastopexy alone on the left side. This would have improved the volume asymmetry but potentially exaggerated shape asymmetry. Alternatively, she could have chosen reduction of the left breast by means of liposuction and some direct tissue excision to equalize the volume followed by bilateral augmentation with the same implant as in the right side and mastopexy [5]. She opted for the second option along with some axillary liposuction.

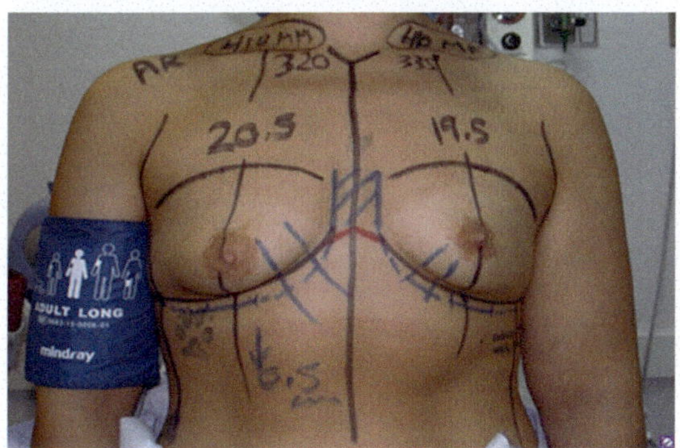

Fig. 5.6

After trying on sizers on the right side, an implant with about 4.0 cm of projection and 300 cc gave her the best volume symmetry (Fig. 5.9). Accordingly, a 310-cc smooth, round, low-profile responsive gel implant with x, y, z of 12/12/4 cm was selected for both sides to achieve upper pole fullness. Responsive gel was chosen to minimize the risk of waterfall deformity, which can occur with the more cohesive implants in the setting of significant volume of glandular tissue in the lower pole.

During the surgery, the reduction of the left breast was done with liposuction removing 225 cc. This reduced the volume asymmetry significantly. After bilateral submuscular augmentation with the same implants, she was still a little bigger on the left side. Further volume adjustment was performed during mastopexy, removing another 40 gm of tissue.

Examination 10 months postoperatively showed relatively good shape and volume asymmetry (Fig. 5.10). Note that she still has some residual pigmented areolar skin along the vertical limb of the breasts that was preserved in order to minimize tension during skin closure.

Secondary Cases with a Large Implant Pocket/Implant Malposition

The imbalance between the mass effect of implants and strength of surrounding supporting structures can wreak havocs, causing secondary deformities and implant malposition. This can happen in patients with poor ligamentous and skin qualities (e.g., postpartum, aging, post weight loss), in patients with implants heavier than what their tissues can support, in patients seeking implant downsizing, and when the surgeon over-dissects the pocket. The remedy for all of these is to regain control of the pocket dimensions and reduce the stress on the surrounding tissues. This may require additional soft-tissue reinforcement.

Whether dealing with a downsizing case where the existing breast pocket is too large for the new smaller implant or the patient has

Fig. 5.7

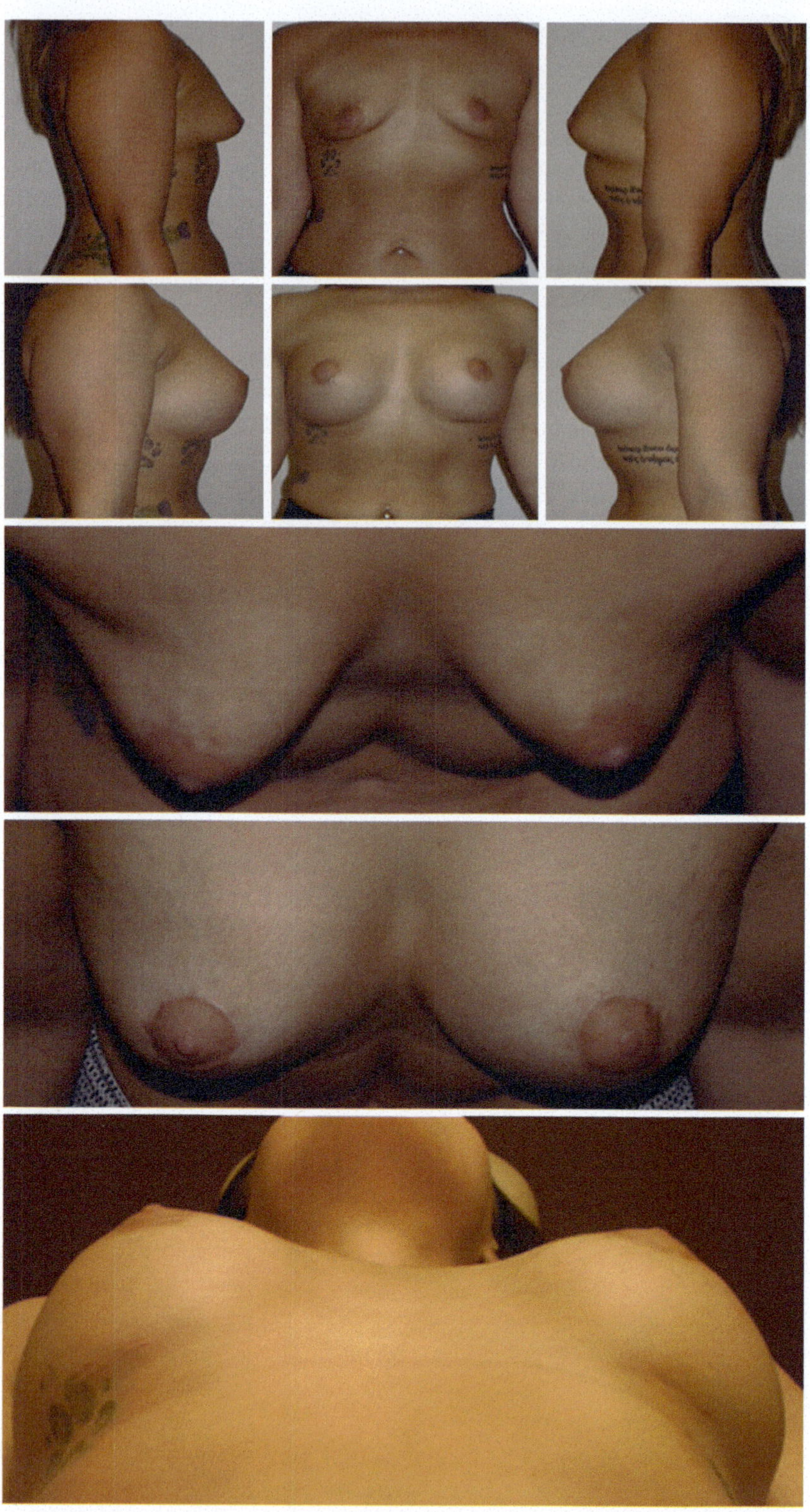

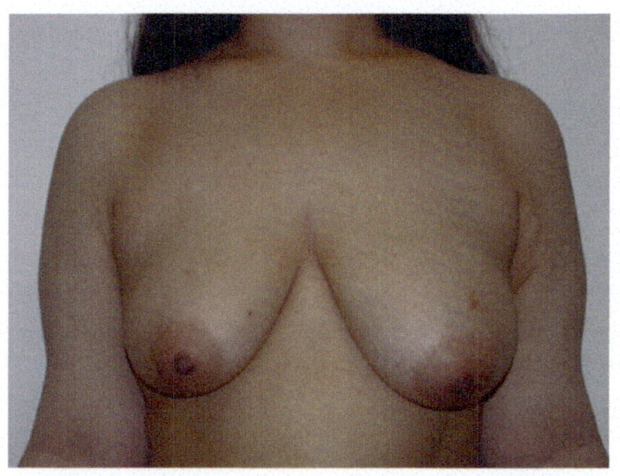

Fig. 5.8

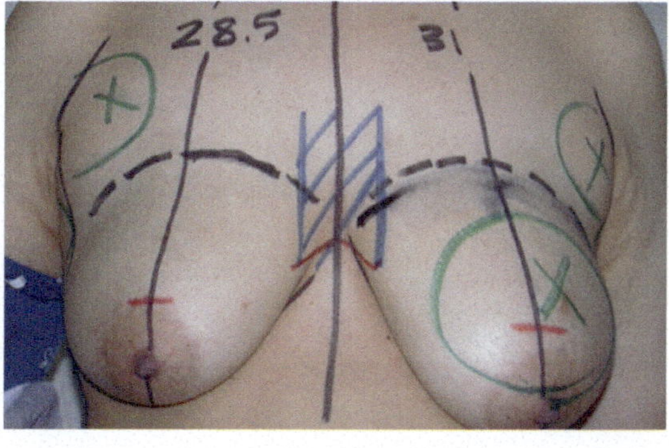

Fig. 5.9

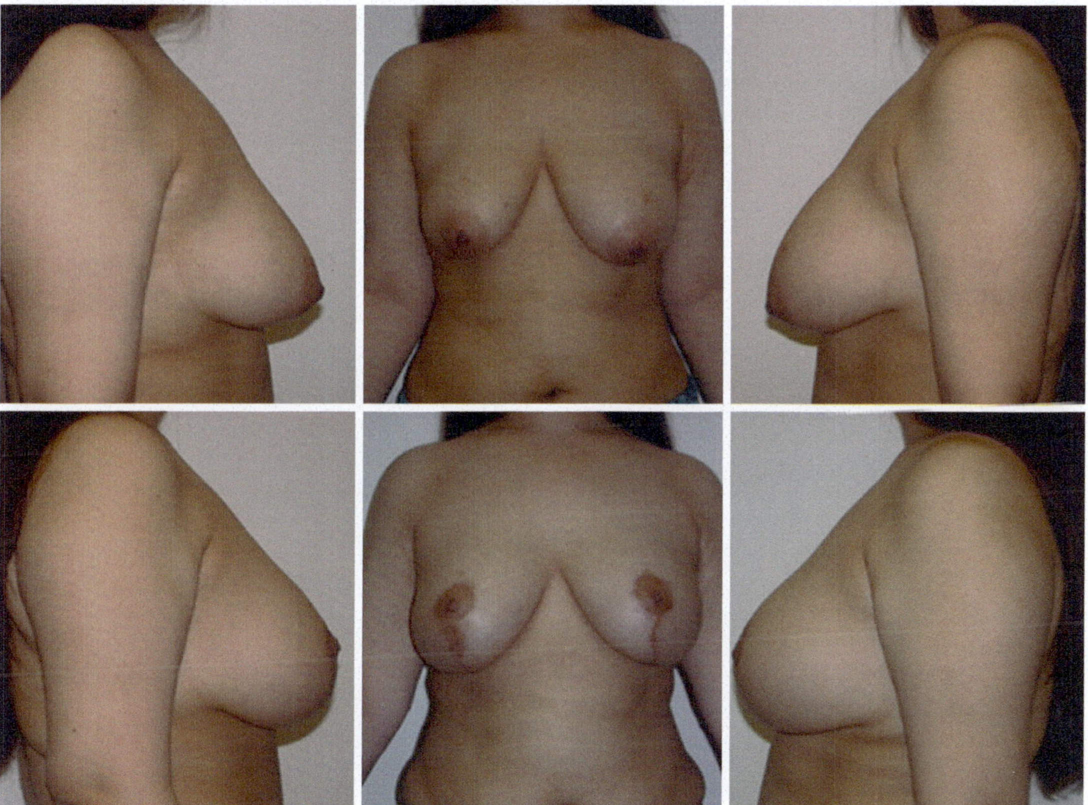

Fig. 5.10

developed malposition due to overstretched pocket, the treatment approach is the same. The safest and most predictable way to deal with this dilemma is to proceed in a two-step fashion by first removing the previous implants and allowing an "implant holiday" until several months later. This allows for contraction of pocket and soft tissue, thus making the creation of sufficiently tight pockets for the new implant possible. In addition, the removal of the implant allows for a more accurate preoperative sizing if implant size or shape change is desired. If the existing implant is saline, the surgeon can deflate the implant and achieve the same goals. However, this approach requires the patient's acceptance for a delayed augmentation. Alternatively, the pocket adjustments can be done in one operation in an algorithmic approach [6].

Case Analysis

The patient is a 29-year-old female who presented for implant revision surgery. She had undergone bilateral submuscular augmentation with 350-cc saline implants after which she had two pregnancies. Postpartum, she developed soft-tissue atrophy with bottoming out of her implant with lateral malposition given her smooth implant and weaker surrounding soft tissue. She wanted to have implant exchange, with slightly larger gel implants with more upper pole fullness and no lateral malposition.

Her examination showed pseudoptotic breasts with soft-tissue atrophy and loss of upper pole fullness and lateral malposition (Fig. 5.11).

In preparation for surgery, her saline implants were deflated in the office under local anesthesia (Fig. 5.12). Three months later, she underwent bilateral augmentation in the same, but contracted,

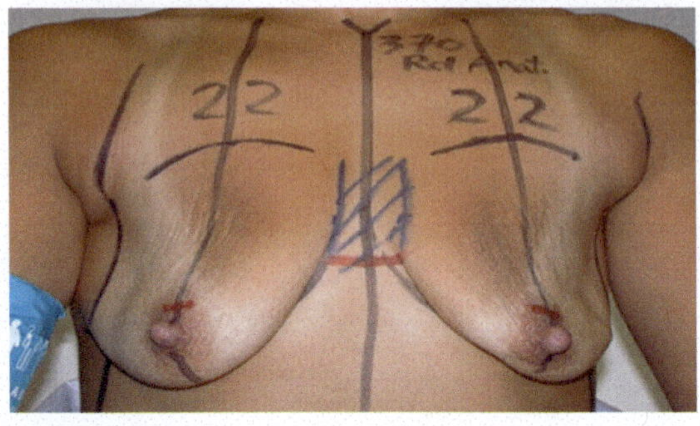

Fig. 5.12

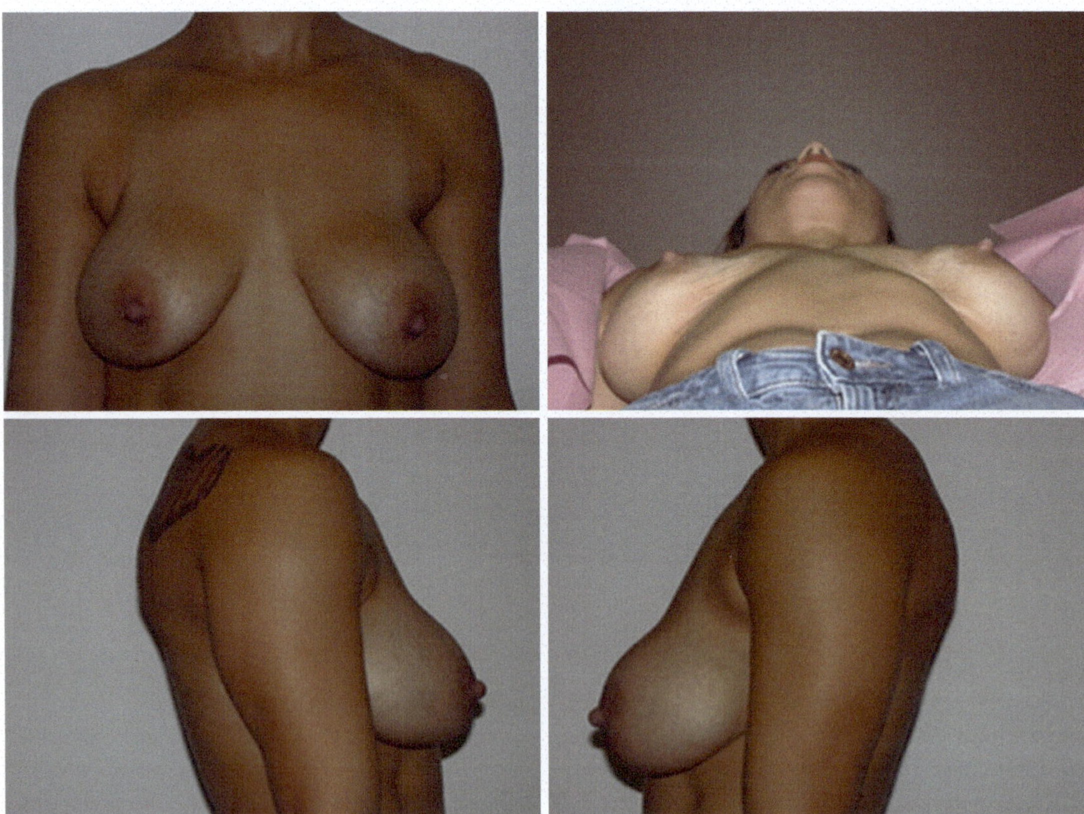

Fig. 5.11

pocket using textured round-base, tear-shaped implants (375-cc 11.9/11.9/5.7 cm) for better pocket stability and mastopexy. Alternatively, smooth, round implants could have been used with possible reinforcement of the pocket with acellular dermal matrix (ADM) or mesh, if necessary.

Her postoperative examination at 1 year showed improved balance in her breast proportions with upper pole fullness, skin envelope reduction, and excellent pocket control (Fig. 5.13).

Correction of Malposition in One Operation: An Algorithmic Approach

As discussed in Chap. 1, the breast is supported and shaped by a system of adhesion zones (circumammary ligaments) and a supportive fascial system (SFS and Cooper's ligament). Furthermore, the smooth implants have a tendency to follow gravity, migrating laterally when laying down and inferiorly when standing. The

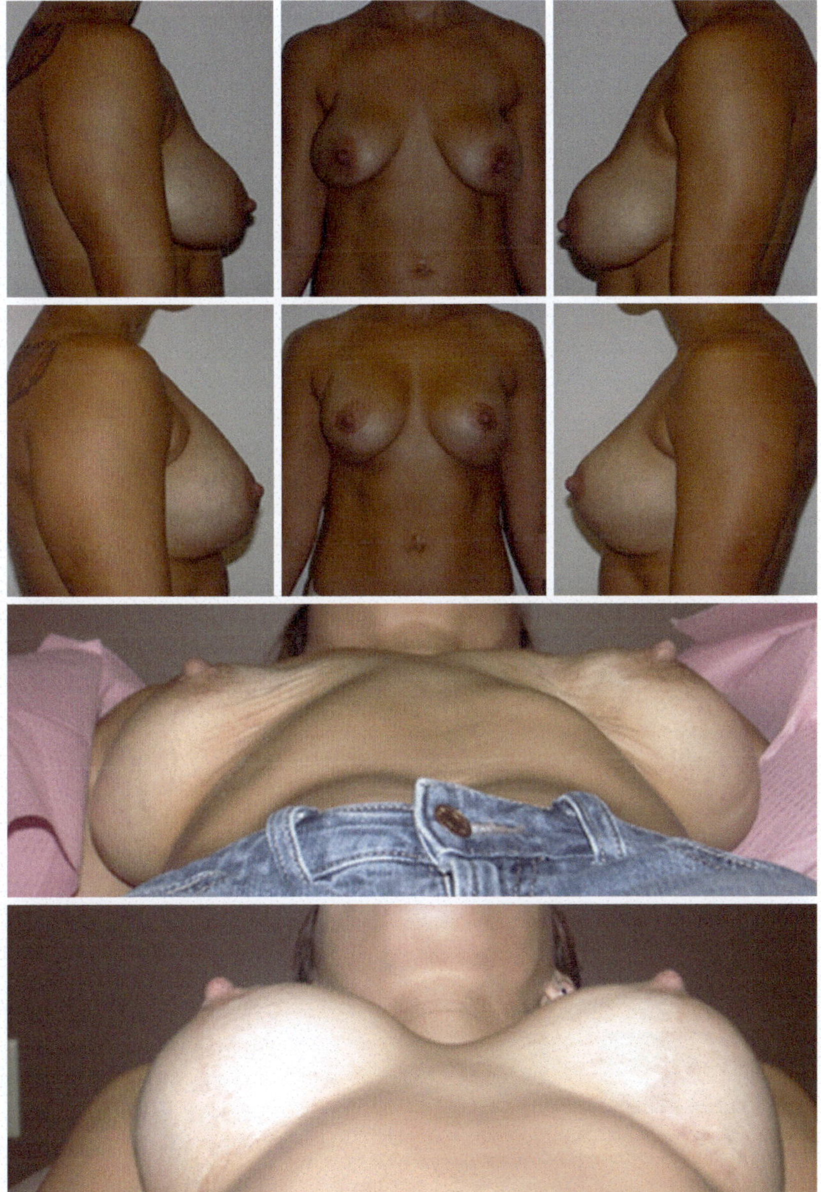

Fig. 5.13

weaker the supportive infrastructure of the breast and the heavier the implant, the higher is the risk for malposition. The occurrence of malposition indicates that the ecosystem in which the implant resides can no longer provide a favorable supportive environment to withstand the weight of the implant. This results in uncontrolled tissue expansion of the internal and external tissues surrounding the pocket. The management, therefore, requires a different thinking. It should be noted that even a textured implant with its better coefficient of friction can behave like a smooth implant, especially if surrounded by double capsule.

In dealing with excess capsular tissues, one should ask the following question: Is the capsule the "foe or friend"? If it is "foe," it should be discarded, but if it is "friend," it can be used to our advantage.

We address malposition in an algorithmic approach (Fig. 5.14) consisting of five components: (1) dual-plane reinforcement capsular flaps (CF) to revise the implant pocket; (2) thermal capsular manipulation to close off dead space and reinforce the repair; (3) implant replacement with a textured device to reduce implant migration/displacement (see Chap. 1 for factors influencing friction and pocket stability, $F = \mu N$) or a smooth device with lateral/inferior pocket reinforcement using mesh or ADM [4, 7]; (4) continuous use of a supportive bra for 6 months to reduce tension laterally and inferiorly while the internal pocket repair is healing; and (5) for recurrent malposition, perform all of the above with addition of mesh or ADM for reinforcement regardless of the surface of implant.

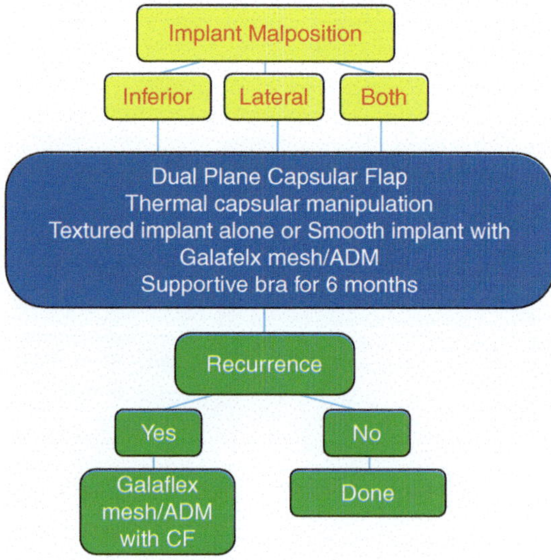

Fig. 5.14 Our algorithm for correction of lateral or inferior implant malposition

Operative Techniques

Preoperatively, during the biodimensional planning, we select the appropriate shape and size of implant to correspond to the new dimensions of the desired pocket based on the patient's anatomy and wishes. Following are operative techniques to address the lateral and inferior implant malposition.

For Lateral Malposition

During the preoperative marking, the lateral extent of the pocket (*X* of the implant) and the superior extent of the pocket (*Y* of the implant) are drawn with the patient in standing position. During the surgery and after pocket exposure, the lateral line is transposed to the lateral capsule using a hypodermic needle transcutaneously (Fig. 5.15a).

Then, this line is further transposed onto the lateral chest wall (posterior capsule) as the desired lateral extent of pocket (Fig. 5.15b). The pocket width is further verified by measuring the desired width of the pocket internally with a ruler (Fig. 5.16a). A laterally based posterior CF is designed in a rectangular fashion with the base (axis of rotation) at the desired lateral extent of the pocket (the *X* of implant) and its length equal to the vertical height of the pocket (the *Y* of the implant). The sides of the rectangle measure 3–4 cm and are medial to the base. The flap area is hydrodissected with dilute local anesthesia, capsulotomies on the three sides of the CF are made, and the flap is raised off the anterior chest wall to the hinge point. This includes the serratus fascia (Fig. 5.16c).

A separate capsulotomy is then made along the line drawn from the previously transposed

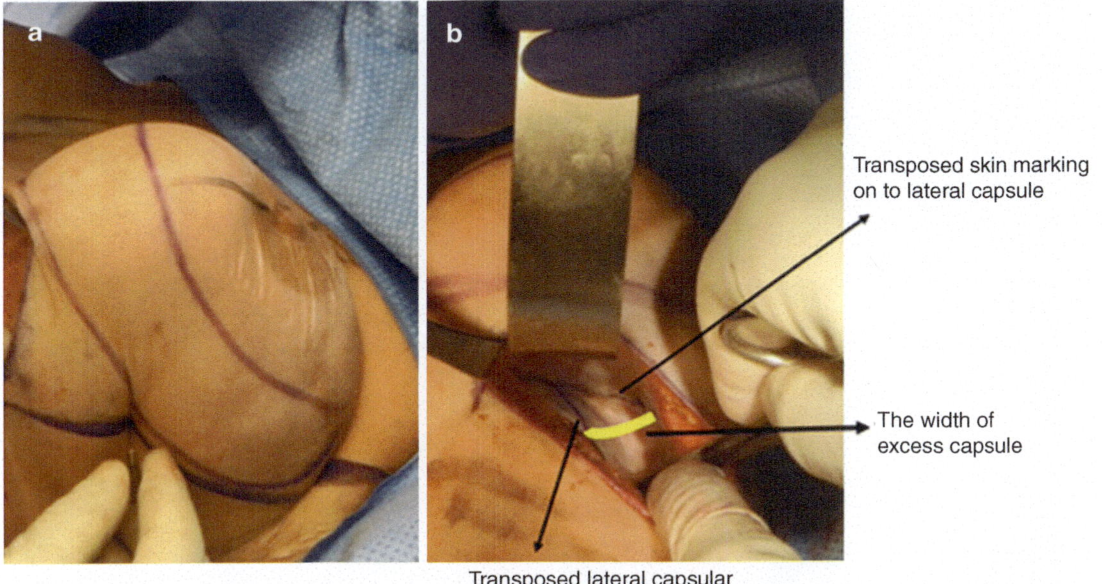

Fig. 5.15 (**a**) Transposition of the lateral breast marking corresponding to the width (*X*) of the implant to the lateral capsule using a hypodermic needle. (**b**) Internal markings of the transposed lateral breast skin marking (the *X*) on to the lateral and posterior capsules and the intervening excess capsule (yellow marking)

cutaneous lateral pocket line onto the lateral capsule. The thermal contraction with monopolar cautery (Marina Medical) is used to shrink the intervening excess capsule between the base of the lateral CF and lateral capsulotomy site of lateral capsule (Fig. 5.16b). This will not only further narrow the pocket but also encourages the adherence of the two interposing capsular layers. The lead edge of the CF and superior lip of the lateral capsulotomy are then sutured together with multiple figure-of-eight braided nylon sutures (0-Neurolon) with care to oppose raw surfaces to promote healing (Fig. 5.16d). This completes the creation of dual-plane CF (Fig. 5.17). It is important to note that the suture line is away from the point of maximal tension. A drain is placed laterally, the pocket is irrigated with triple antibiotics (see Chap. 1), and the implant is inserted with no touch technique using a sleeve.

For Inferior Malposition

The new ideal IMF is marked preoperatively. In many instances, this coincides with the previous incision scar, which is now riding higher on the inferior pole. If the old scar is not at the proper location, the new incision is made at the desired location based on the algorithms described in Chap. 1. After the skin incision is made, the pericapsular dissection is made anteriorly to the inferior edge of the pectoralis major muscle (in the subpectoral pocket) or for 5 cm (in the prepectoral pocket), at which time a capsulotomy is made and the implant is removed. At this point, a decision is made as to whether we make an inferiorly based posterior CF or an inferiorly based anterior CF based on the quality of anterior capsule and ease of raising the posterior capsule (Figs. 5.18 and 5.19). If an inferiorly based anterior CF is planned, a counter capsulotomy is made on the posterior capsule corresponding to the new IMF based on the skin incision. Alternatively, if an inferiorly based posterior CF is planned due to poor quality of the anterior capsule, a mark is made along the posterior capsule corresponding to the new IMF (same as skin incision). This will be the axis of rotation for the inferiorly based posterior CF. A second line is marked 2–3 cm superior and parallel to the first line. This becomes the superior edge of the CF,

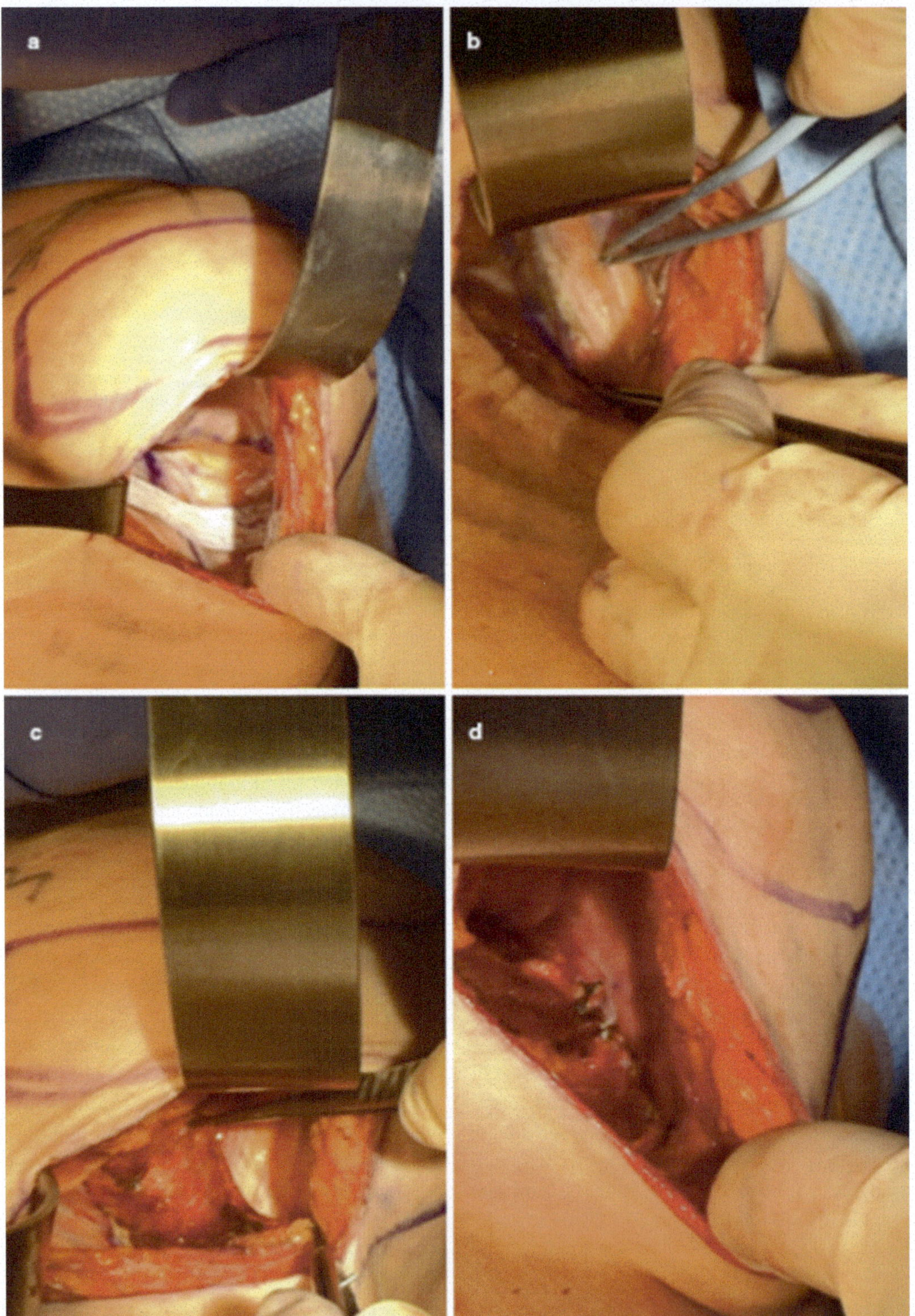

Fig. 5.16 (**a**) Verification of desired pocket width in accordance with the *X* of the implant. (**b**) Thermal contraction of the excess lateral capsule to reduce the dead space and encourage adhesion. (**c**) Laterally based CF is raised that includes serratus fascia for vascularity. (**d**) The laterally based CF is sutured to lateral capsulotomy made at the site of transposed skin marking. This keeps the suture line away from the point of maximum tension

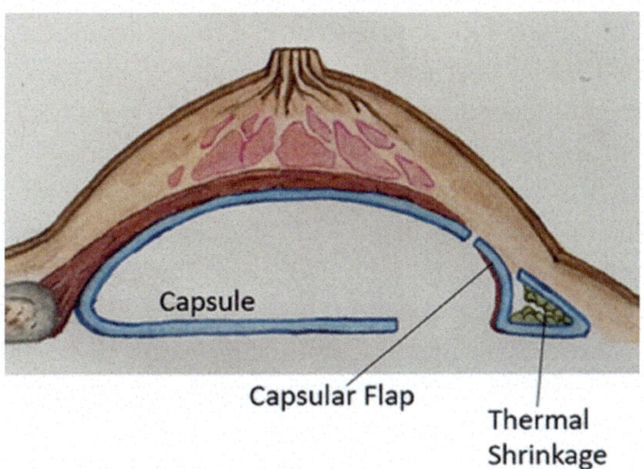

Fig. 5.17 Schematic representation of the laterally based CF to correct lateral implant malposition

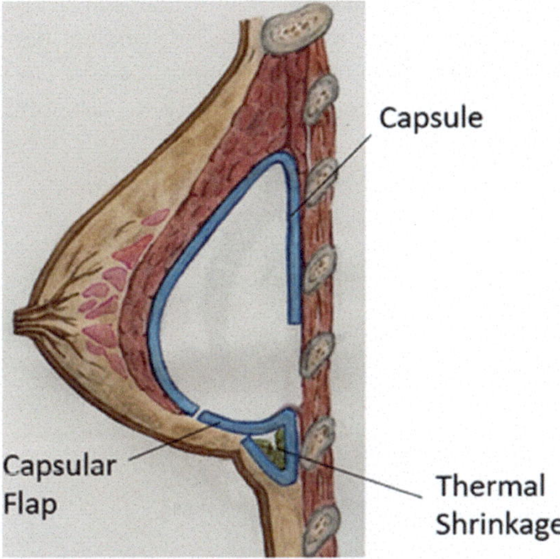

Fig. 5.18 Inferiorly based posterior capsular flap

where after hydrodissection, a capsulotomy is made parallel to the entire length of IMF. The CF is then raised to the new IMF line. The excess capsule between the base of CF and existing fold below the level of skin incision is then treated with the thermal contraction technique, as outlined above. This also encourages the adherence of the two surfaces in this potential dead space. Any extra CF tissue (anterior or posterior) is further folded onto itself to fill this dead space and help create a stronger shelf. The lead edge of the CF and the opposing capsulotomy sites are then sutured together with multiple figure-of-eight braided nylon sutures (0-Neurolon sutures), taking care to oppose raw surfaces to promote healing. It is important to note that the suture line is away from the point of maximal tension.

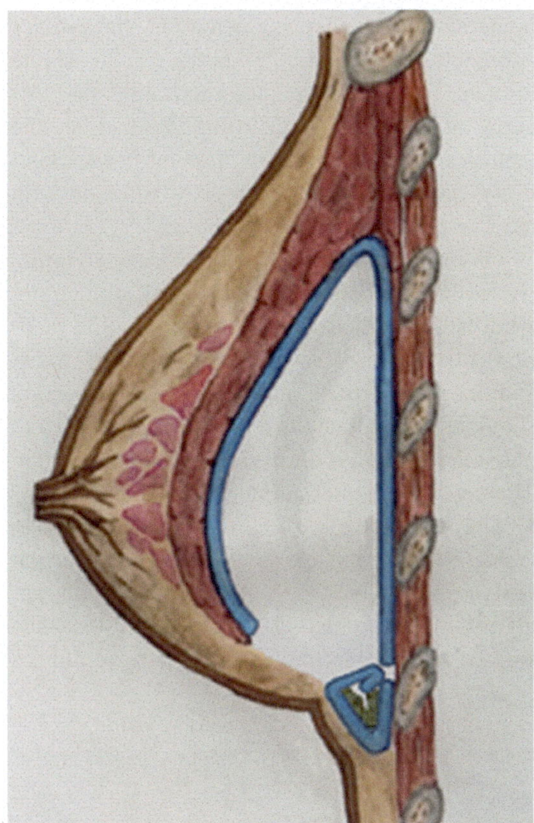

Fig. 5.19 Inferiorly based anterior capsular flap

For Correction of Recurrent Lateral and Inferior Malposition

Strategy for treatment of recurrent malposition cases is the same except in these patients; the tissues have proven to lack adequate inherent strength to support the implant despite the repair with CF. Hence, reinforcement of repair with either ADM or Galaflex scaffold (Galatea Surgical, Inc., Lexington, MA) is required. In these situations, the same algorithmic steps are followed as discussed above with the addition of alloplastic materials as onlay grafts.

Case Analysis

A 34-year-old G1P1 female presented for implant exchange surgery and a lift. She had undergone bilateral submuscular augmentation via axillary approach with 330-cc smooth, round saline implants several years before. Later, she lost body fat through weight lifting. With time, she then developed asymmetry, implant border visibility, and malposition with dissatisfaction with the shape and volume of her breasts.

On examination, she had significant asymmetry, with the left breast displaced inferolaterally while standing and laterally in the supine position (Fig. 5.20). Skeletally, she had pectus excavatum, visible ribs, and scoliosis, with right shoulder higher than the left. She had visible and palpable rippling with a visible implant border. There was wide intermammary distance.

She was given two options. The first was to deflate the implants and revise later. The second option was a one-stage surgery based on our algorithm. She opted for the latter. Since she wanted less visible implants and less rippling, a tall-height 450-cc tear-shaped implant (with *x*/*y*/*z* of 13/14/5 cm) was recommended. She was also recommended fat injection for implant periphery, but she refused.

The patient underwent bilateral inferior and lateral capsular flaps with the use of textured implants. Note that the IMF incisions were made at the desired location based on the width of implant, with the goal of raising the left IMF by 1.5 cm (Fig. 5.21). Postoperatively, she continued to wear a supportive bra continuously.

One year postoperatively, she demonstrated improved balance to her breasts with less visibility of the implant borders and resolution of malposition. Also, a tall-height implant allowed for more volume in the upper pole, which she lacked before. Note that she still has some implant border visibility due to the paucity of soft-tissue coverage, and fat injection could have been helpful (Fig. 5.22).

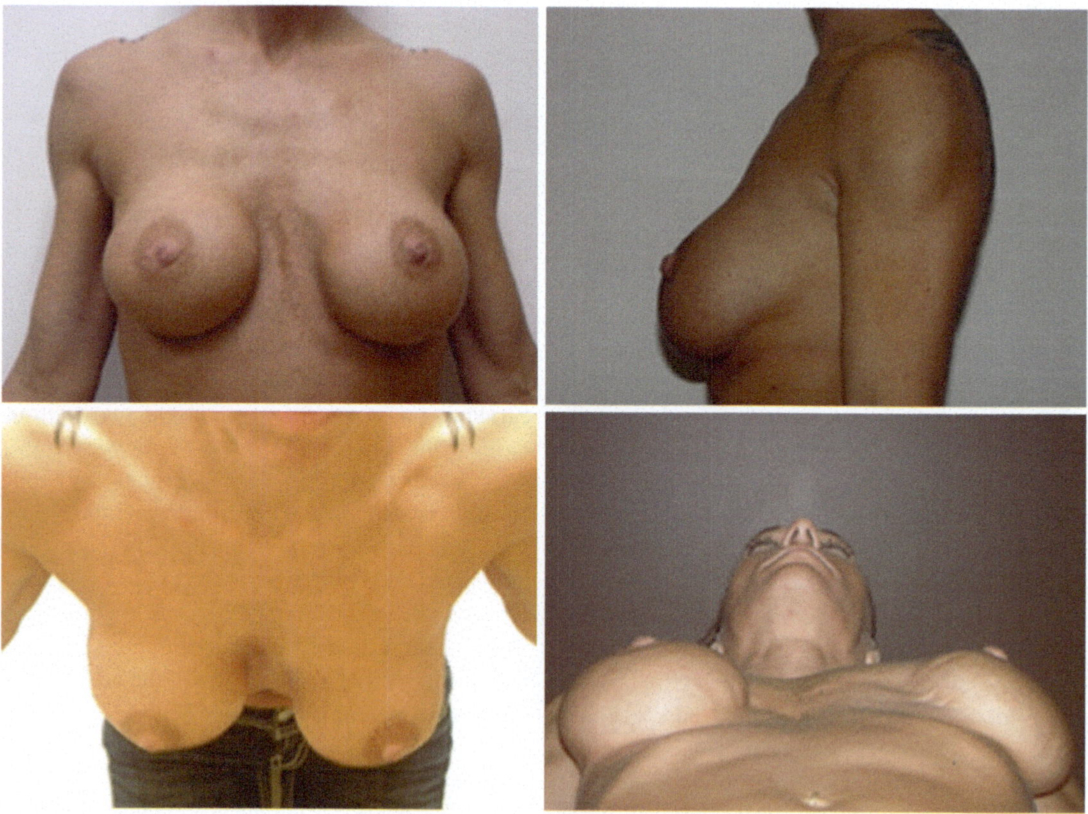

Fig. 5.20

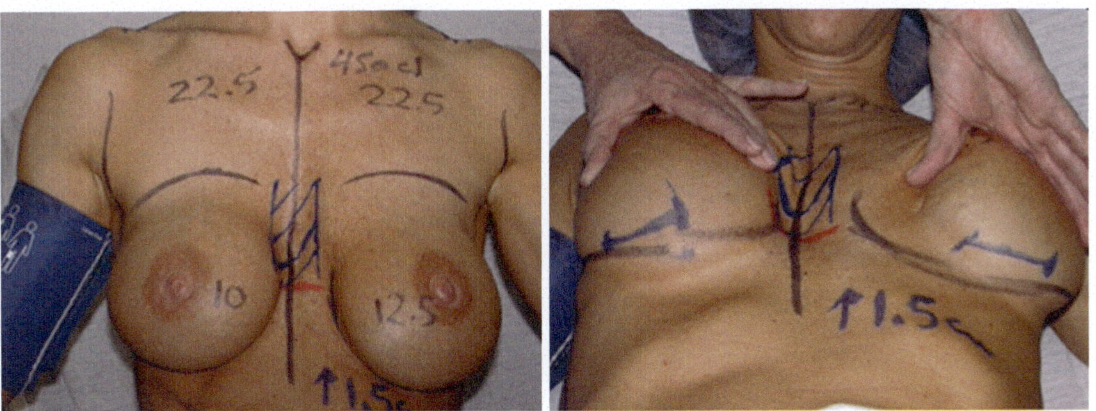

Fig. 5.21

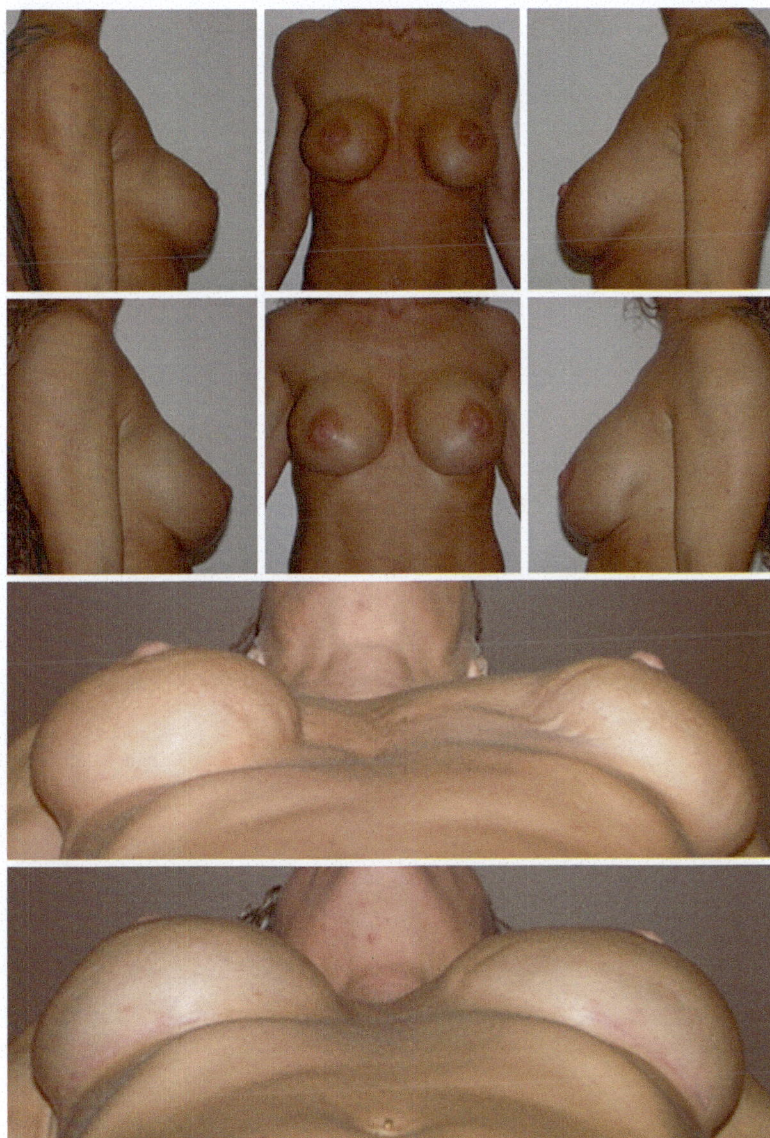

Fig. 5.22

Case Analysis

The patient is a 55-year-old female who presented for breast augmentation after massive weight loss. She had previously undergone breast reduction (Fig. 5.23a). She was augmented with a smooth, round implant and mastopexy. She developed malposition inferiorly and laterally (Fig. 5.23b). Based on our algorithm, she underwent pocket correction with lateral and inferior capsular flaps using textured implants. This was complicated by recurrent malposition as before and stretching of the lower poles (Fig. 5.23c). Therefore, based on our algorithm, since she had failed the above treatment once, her tissue was proven to lack the ability to withstand the forces of gravity. In addition, intraoperatively, we noted that she had developed double capsules, and the implants were behaving like smooth implants. Hence, we planned on repeating the capsular flaps along with reverse abdominoplasty to address some upper abdominal laxity and create a stronger shelf for the smooth implants to sit on. The new IMF was further reinforced with Galaflex mesh (Fig. 5.23d).

In combining reverse abdominoplasty with the other steps to create stable fold, IMF fold was marked to allow about 10 cm of distance from nipple downward, which corresponded to the previous IMF scar. The reverse abdominoplasty was estimated preoperatively and verified intraoperatively. Note the amount of skin excision and securing of the skin edge to the desired fold location by suturing SFS to the deep fascia using multiple 0-Neurolon sutures (Fig. 5.24a), reinforcement of the fold and lateral capsular flap with Galaflex mesh as an onlay graft (Fig. 5.24b), and lateral malposition before (Fig. 5.24c) and after correction (Fig. 5.24d).

Postoperatively, she continued to wear a supportive bra and has had excellent stable result for 18 months (Fig. 5.25).

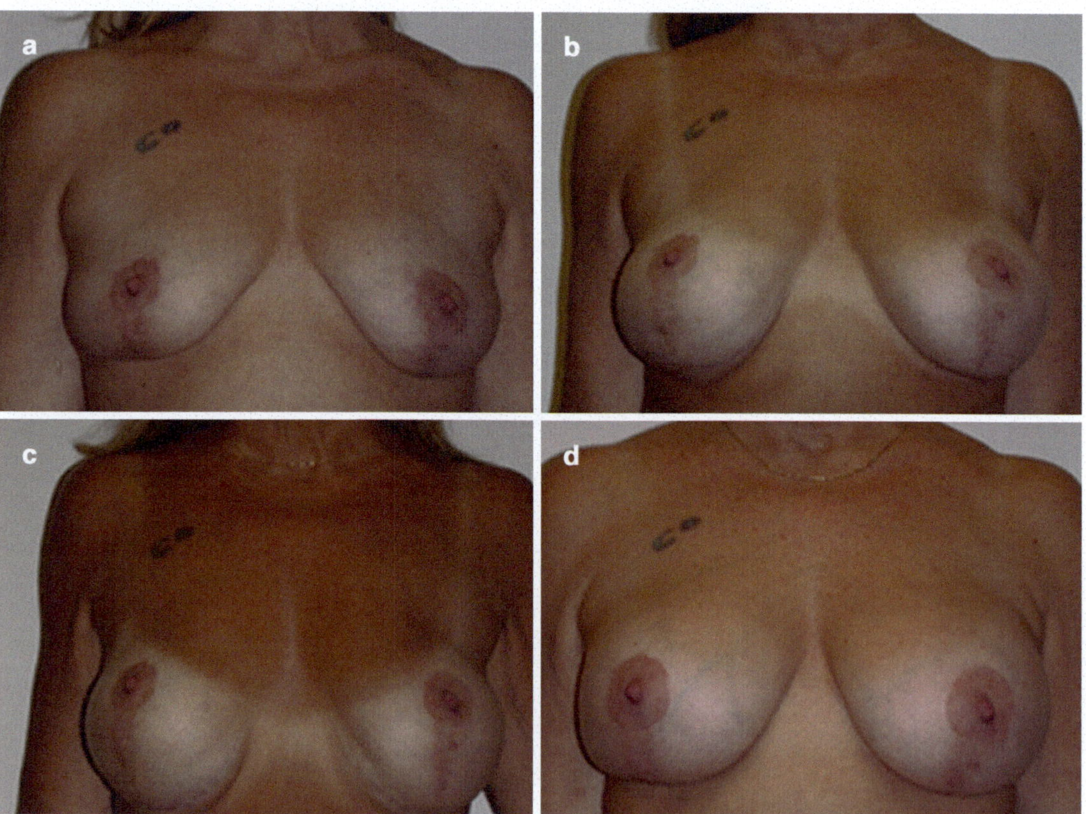

Fig. 5.23

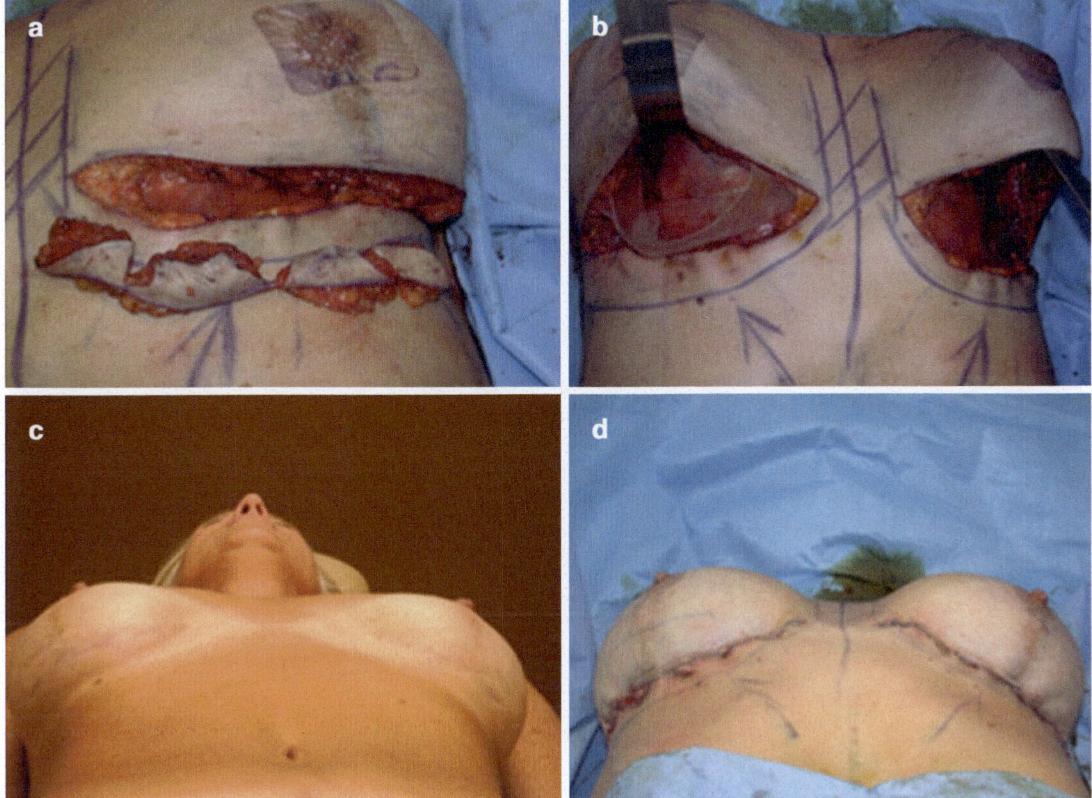

Fig. 5.24

Correction of Pectoralis Disruption

This deformity occurs from overzealous release of origin of pectoralis major muscle from the sternum while creating a dual-plane pocket. It usually presents itself as an asymmetric medial border of breasts with the loss of the natural silhouette at rest (Fig. 5.26b). When the patient is asked to flex the pectoralis major muscle, the implant moves medially (Fig. 5.26c).

The treatment options include changing the pocket from subpectoral to prepectoral with an attempt to reattach the muscle if the patient qualifies for subfascial augmentation. Alternatively, if the prepectoral pocket is not an option, that is, in a patient who has a paucity of soft tissue, one can attempt to repair the muscle and recreate the medial border of the pocket with the use ADM.

Case Analysis

The patient is a 54-year-old female who presented with asymmetry and misshapen left breast (Fig. 5.27). She had undergone submuscular breast augmentation with textured round implants. Postoperatively, she developed loss of normal medial border of left breast and visible rippling.

On examination, she had visible ribs with a paucity of soft-tissue coverage. As a result, she had visible implant border and rippling. Also, because of adherence of textured implant to the capsule and subsequent loosening of the lower pole tissue, she had visible irregularity in the lower poles. In addition, there was loss of normal medial silhouette of the left breast. On animation, the implant moved superomedially with loss of medial pocket border.

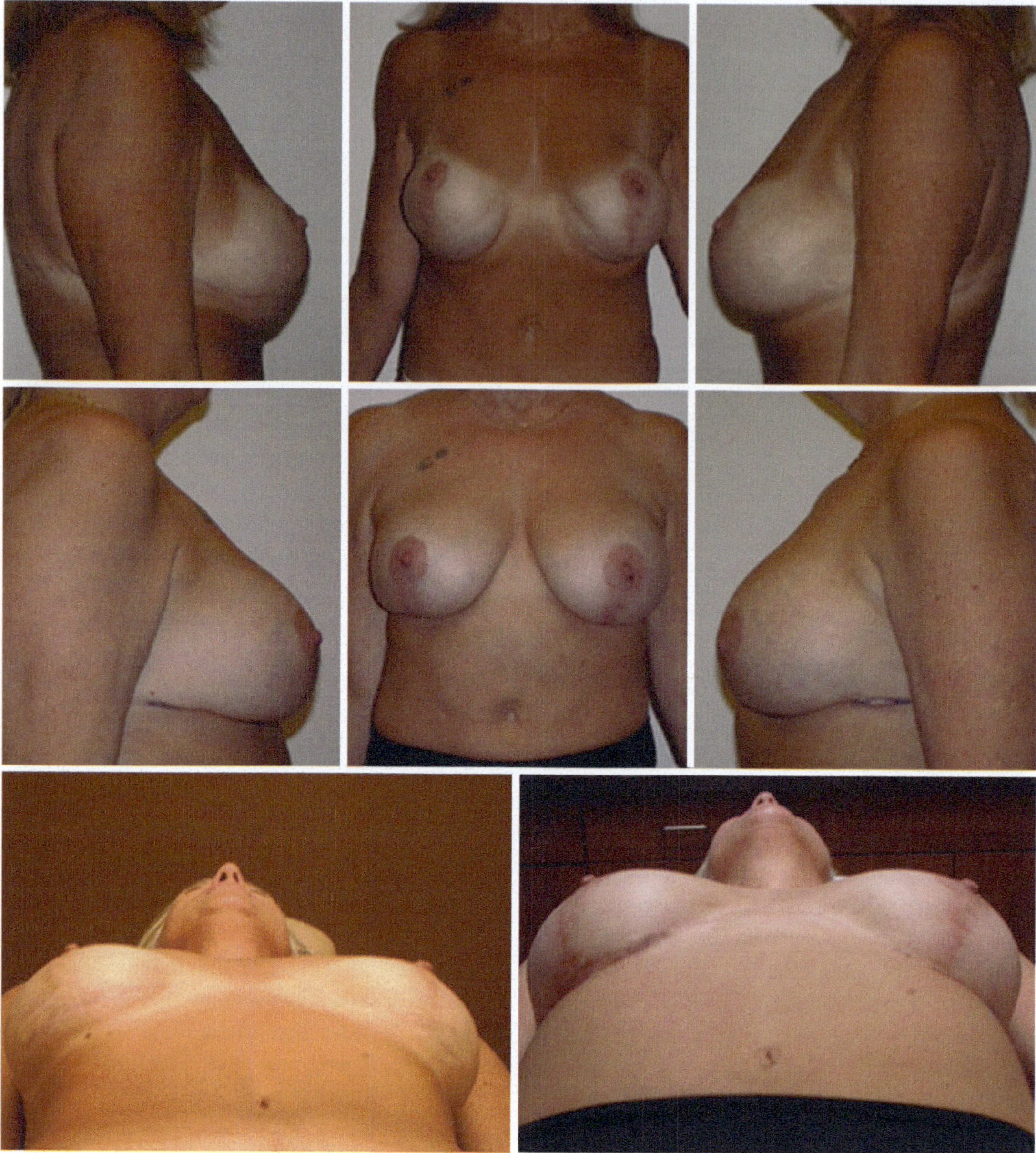

Fig. 5.25

Given the paucity of soft-tissue coverage, the change of pocket to subfascial pocket was not an option. Therefore, reaugmentation in the same pocket was attempted with plans to use ADM to correct the medial border (Fig. 5.28a). This was done by first performing partial capsulectomy where there was tethering in the lower poles. Then, the free inferior and medial borders of the pectoralis major muscle were identified and freed up for 2 cm. The boundaries of bilateral pectoralis muscles were marked on skin. Note the displacement of the medial border of left muscle (Fig. 5.28b). ADM was used to help reestablish the medial attachment of the left muscle and recreate the medial border of the pocket by suturing the ADM to the muscle on one side and the capsule of the medial pocket on the other side. Note the loss of medial border of the left breast before

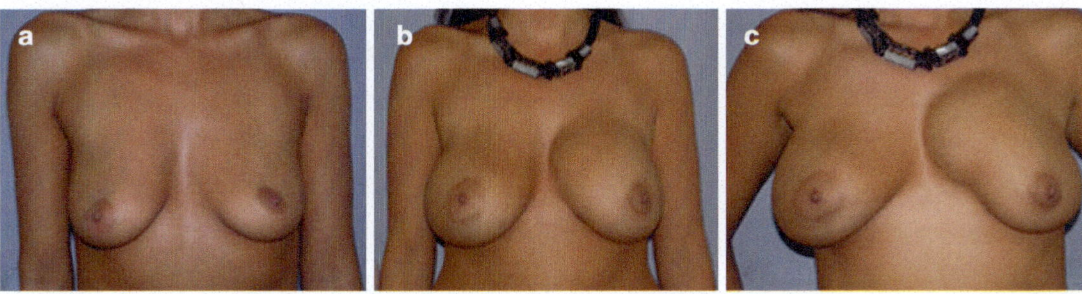

Fig. 5.26

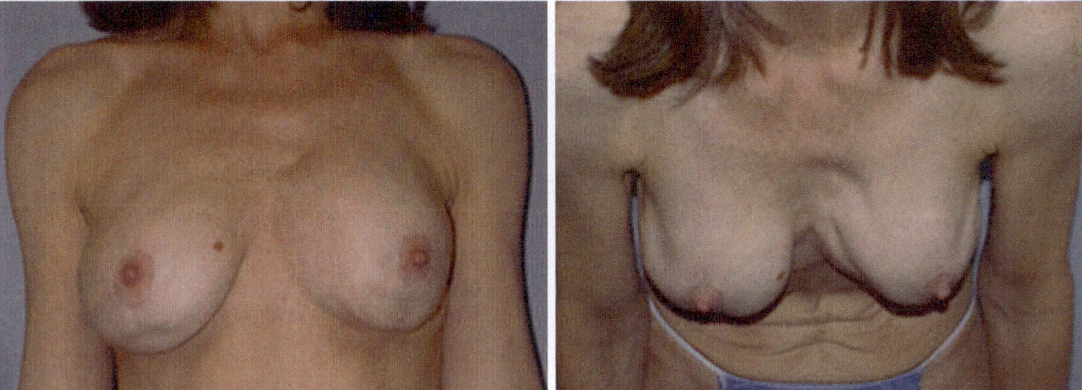

Fig. 5.27

repair (Fig. 5.28c) and after repair (Fig. 5.28d). Smooth round gel implants were then used followed by mastopexy.

Note postoperative stability at 1 year (Fig. 5.29).

Double-Bubble Deformity

The etiologies for double-bubble deformity (DBD) are inadequate release of IMF structures while lowering the IMF in a breast with short lower pole and constricted base (the ligamentous structure maintain its tissue memory), the pistol effect of pectoralis major muscle forming an indentation band over the lower pole of the breast, and the loss of IMF control with the implant dropping below the fold. This patient demonstrates the loss of IMF control and unfavorable pistol effect of pectoralis muscle on animation (Fig. 5.30a–d).

The correction of DBD will depend on the underlying cause. In case of loss of IMF control, the algorithm for inferior malposition in Fig. 5.14 can be used. For other causes, that is, when the muscle plays an unfavorable role, pocket conversion from submuscular to subfascial pocket eliminates the muscle influence and corrects the issue. Alternatively, when the tissue thickness is inadequate for subfascial pocket and/or if a simpler solution is sought, rigotomy of the indented lower pole area and correction of the defect with fat injection provide a good option (see Chap. 3).

Case Analysis

A 40-year-old female presented with postpartum breast atrophy. She underwent bilateral breast augmentation in dual-plane I pocket with textured round, responsive gel implants, 485 cc on the right side and 450 cc on the left side.

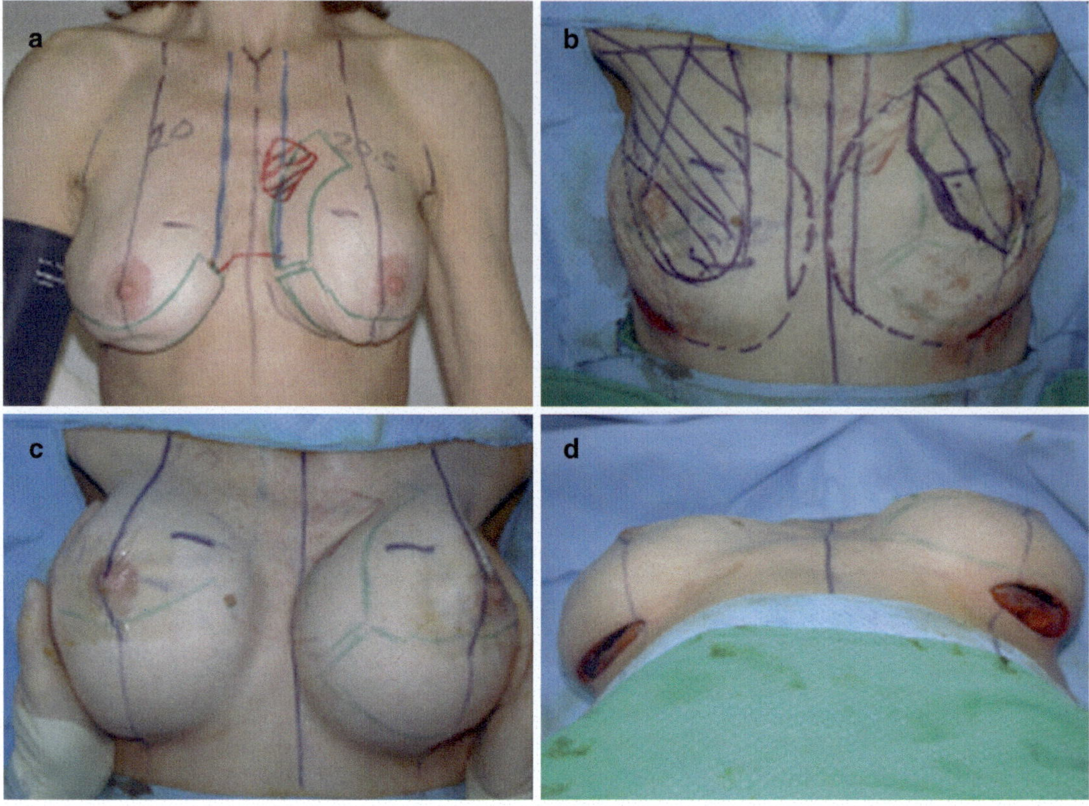

Fig. 5.28

Postoperatively, she developed DBD due to unfavorable muscle activity. In addition, she developed lateral malposition (Fig. 5.31).

She was happy with her overall volume but wished to have more upper pole fullness. Given her adequate upper pole pinch test of more than 2 cm, a change of pocket from submuscular to subfascial pocket was planned to eliminate muscle action. The pectoralis muscle was repaired back down to its origin. In addition, inferior and lateral pocket control was achieved using the algorithm in Fig. 5.14 with capsular flaps. To achieve more upper pole fullness, the same size textured implant with more cohesivity was used (Fig. 5.32).

Note the intraoperative correction of lateral malposition (Fig. 5.33).

Postoperatively, she continued to wear her supportive bra continuously with good stability at 1 year and resolution of DBD and lateral malposition (Fig. 5.34).

Unilateral Breast Reconstruction with Contralateral Breast Post Mastopexy/Reduction Bottoming Out

Achieving breast symmetry when doing unilateral breast reconstruction with an implant in the setting of a contralateral breast ptosis/macromastia is one of the most frustrating situations in breast surgery. The issue is that the implant in a tight pocket surrounded by a tight skin envelope remains higher on the chest with more upper pole projection depending on the profile and cohesivity of the implant used. On the other hand, the contralateral natural breast with its loose tissue and skin envelope will settle after mastopexy/breast reduction, regardless of the technique used with increasing N-IMF distance (bottoming out). This occurs because the supporting structures of the natural breast (SFS, circumammary ligaments, and Cooper's ligaments) have attenuated

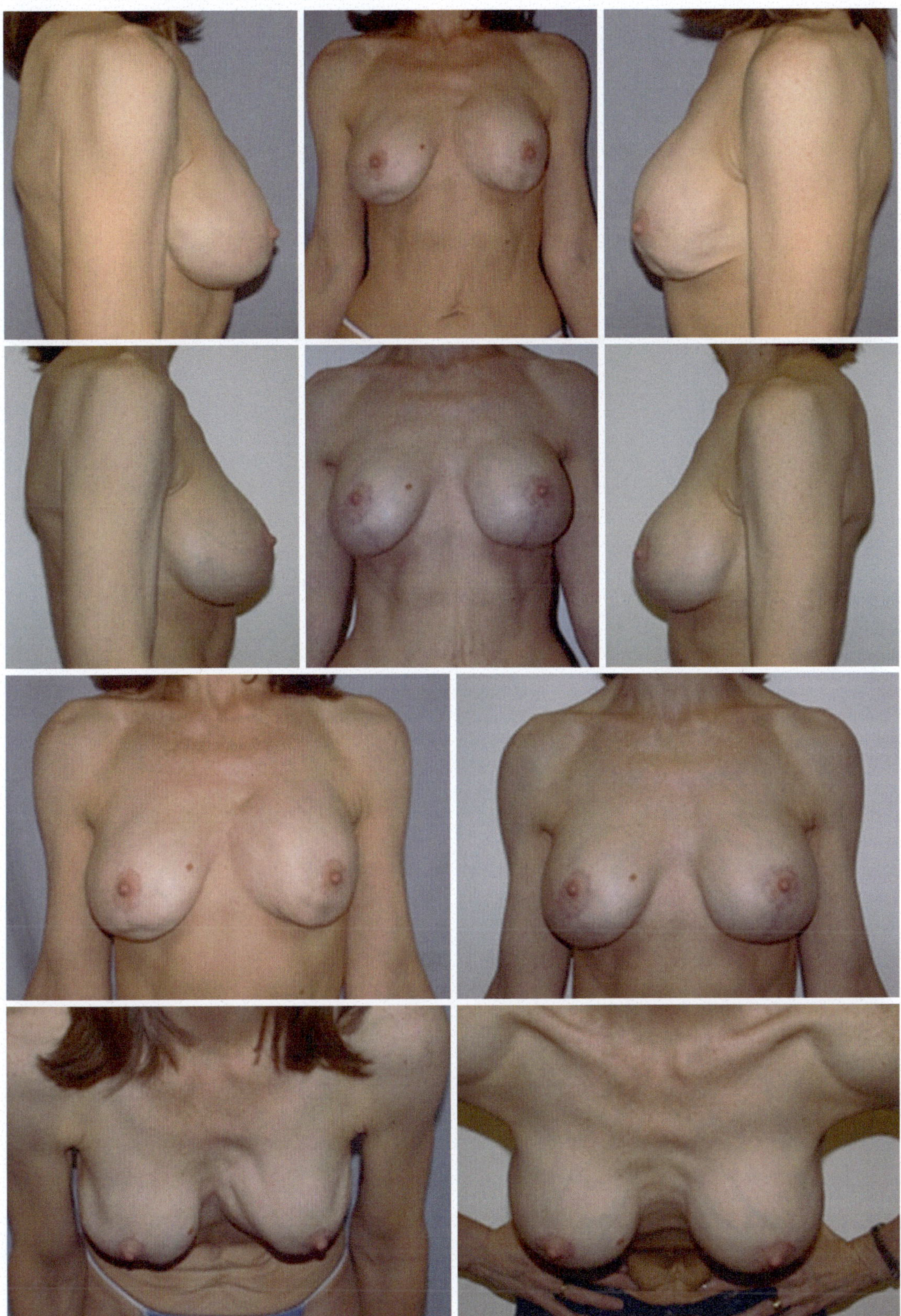

Fig. 5.29

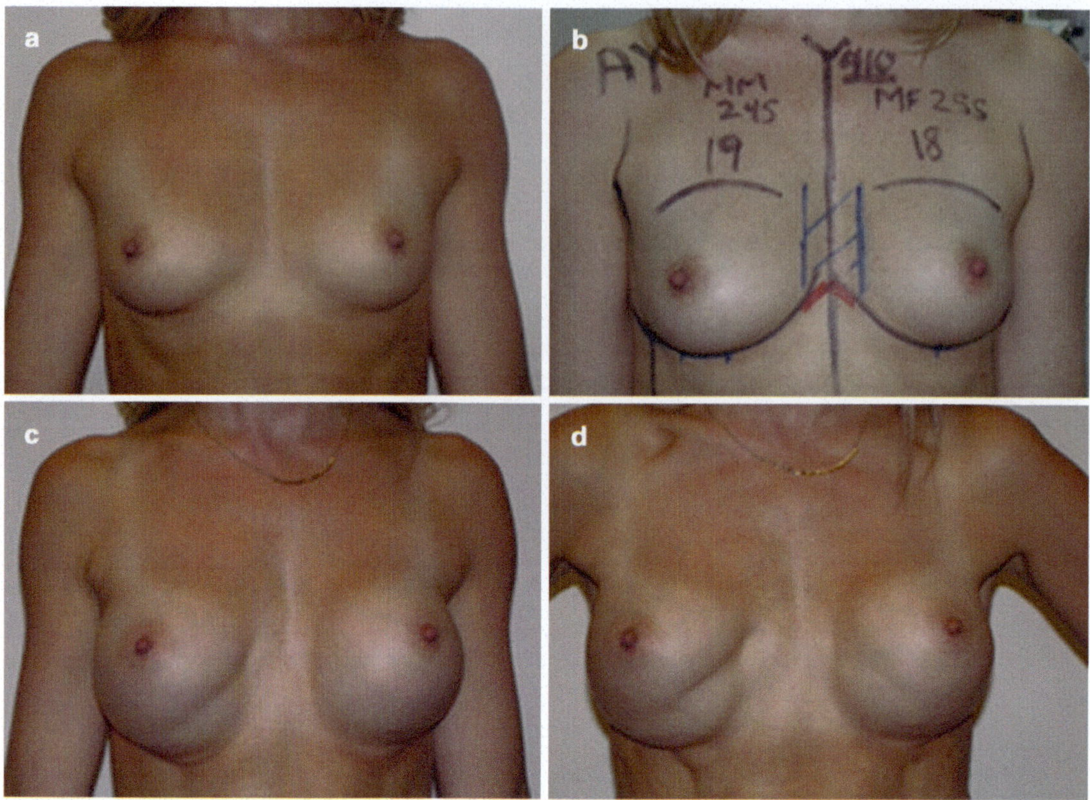

Fig. 5.30 Double-bubble deformity in a patient who underwent submuscular breast augmentation with tear-shaped gel implants. (**a**) Preoperatively. (**b**) Surgical marking with incision made at the existing IMF. (**c**) Double-bubble deformity at rest due to inferior malposition (worse on the right) and persistent memory of IMF ligamentous structure. (**d**) Double-bubble deformity exacerbated with pectoralis animation

and are not strong enough to maintain the desired vertical position established during a lifting procedure. To remedy this problem and maintain lower pole stability, one can use ADM or mesh materials (our preference is Galaflex scaffold mesh) as a sling during mastopexy/reduction surgery. This can help reinforce the weakened supporting structures of the breast and provide some stability in N-IMF distance [8]. To address the asymmetry in the upper pole fullness, consider either a lower profile implant on the reconstructed side or augmentation of the contralateral breast with an implant and/or fat injection.

Case Summary

The patient is a 45-year-old female with a history of symptomatic macromastia who presented with a newly diagnosed right breast cancer (Fig. 5.35). After completing adjuvant chemotherapy, she presented for right breast mastectomy. Given the proximity of the tumor to the nipple, skin-sparing mastectomy and immediate two-stage breast reconstruction with implant were planned in the prepectoral pocket.

Surgically, mastectomy was designed by excising the nipple and de-epithelializing the central excess skin in a smile pattern mastopexy with the superior incision at the Pitanguy point (new nipple location) and the lower incision 8–10 cm above the IMF (Fig. 5.36). The smile pattern mastopexy allows for reduction of both transverse and vertical excess skin while avoiding the Wise pattern skin reduction with the T-junction scar. The de-epithelialized skin is then advanced and secured under the superior skin flap for more thickness. Of note, in case the nipple-areolar complex could be preserved, this technique allows for either inclusion of NAC as part of the dermal flap or be added to the superior flap as a graft. In case of inclusion as part of the dermal flap, a window

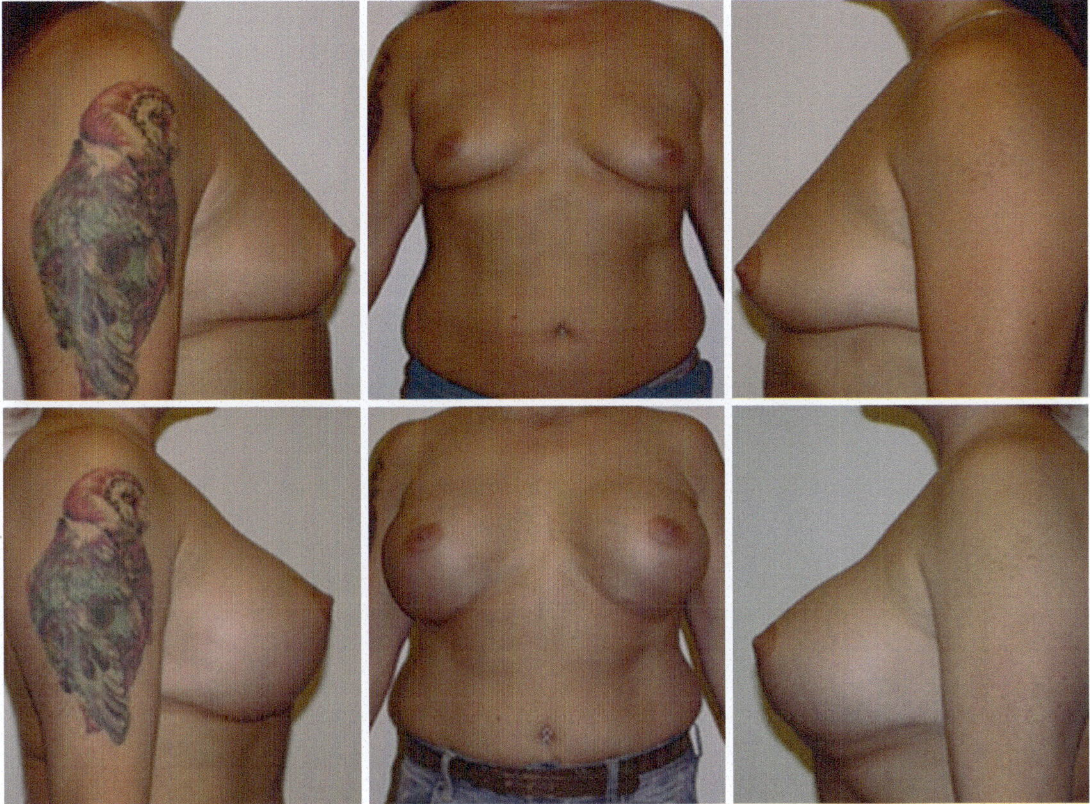

Fig. 5.31

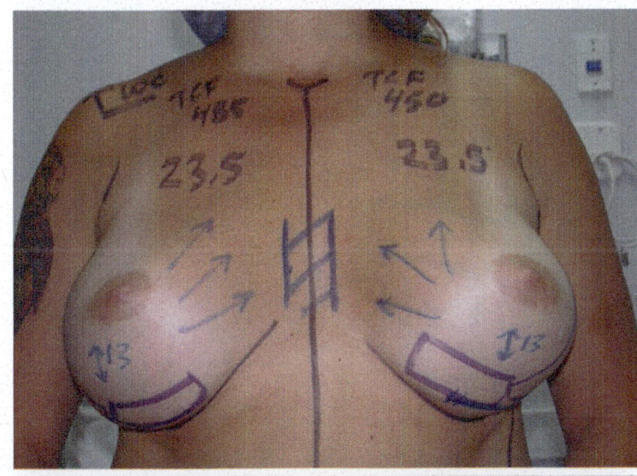

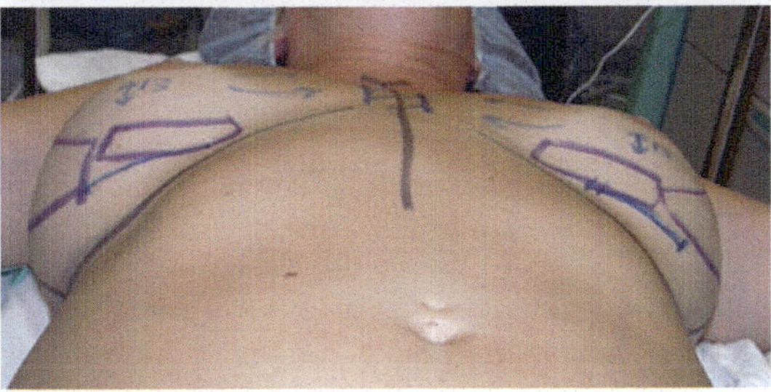

Fig. 5.32

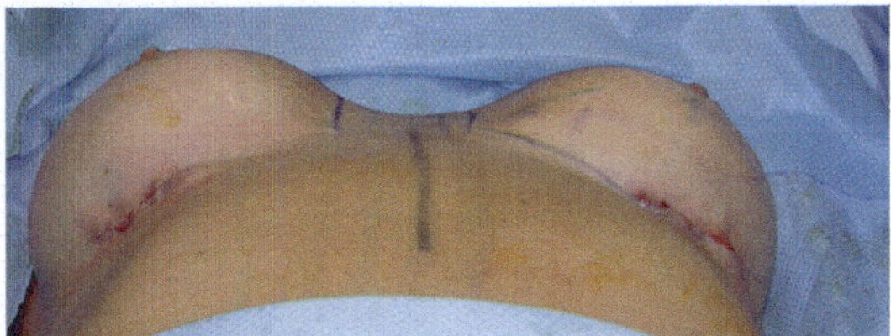

Fig. 5.33

along the supperior incision (Pitanguy point) is created to accomodate the NAC.

Six months later, the patient returned for the stage II reconstruction (Fig. 5.37). The plan was to replace the expander with a 615-cc smooth, round soft touch gel implant and inject the skin envelope with fat injection. For the contralateral side, breast reduction and axillary liposuction were planned. In order to minimize lower pole bottoming out, Galaflex mesh was used as an internal sling to support the inferior pedicle.

A technical note about the use of this mesh is that the tension established at the time of opera-

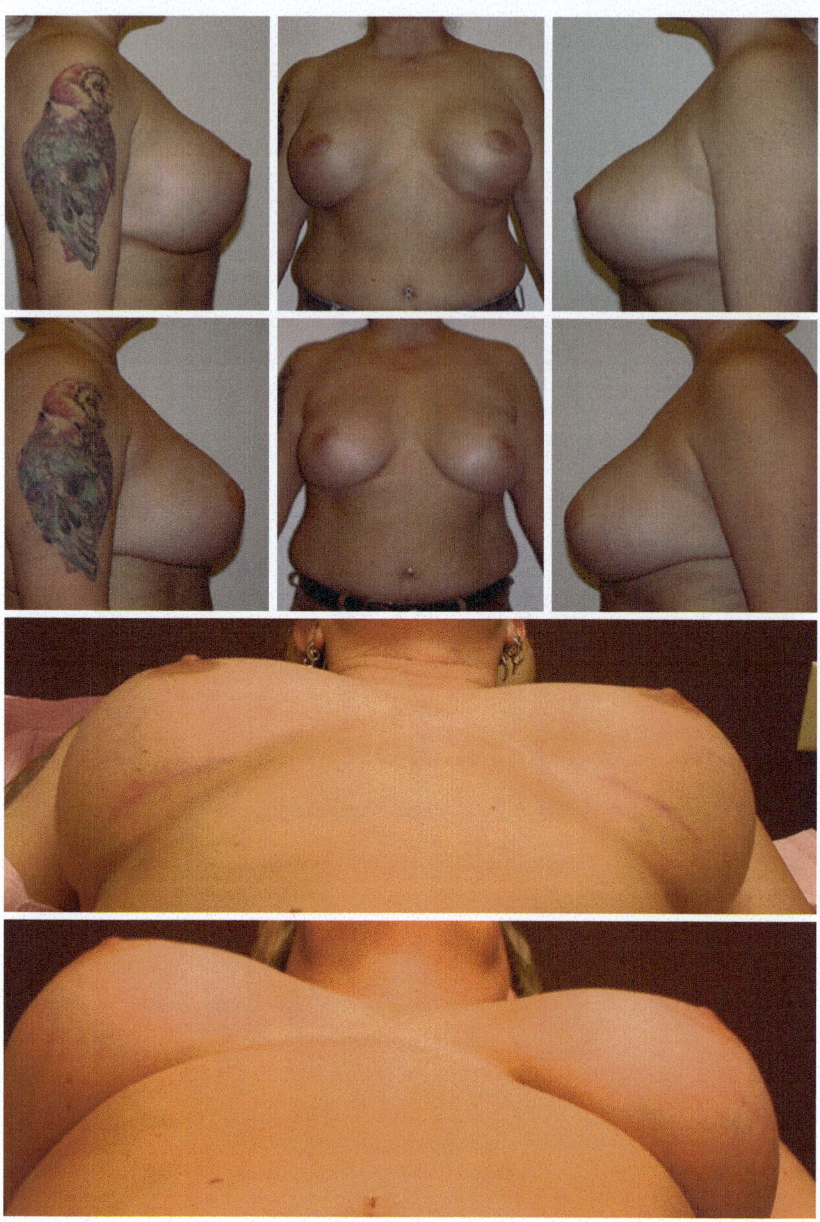

Fig. 5.34

tion must be set with the patient in the sitting position with the lower pole at the desired location to match the contralateral side. There will be no significant settling with time. Note also that the lower border of the mesh is about 1 cm above the IMF incision to avoid exposure in case of T-junction dehiscence (Fig. 5.38).

At 9 months, she continues to enjoy very good symmetry of lower poles as well as an overall good cosmetic outcome (Fig. 5.39).

Symmastia

Symmastia presents one of the most challenging situations in revision breast surgery. The underlying etiology is the loss of medial border of the breast by either over releasing the pectoralis muscle in the subpectoral pocket or medial boundary of the breast in the prepectoral pocket. The solutions are pocket change, neo-pocket creation using the pectoralis fascia, and/or exist-

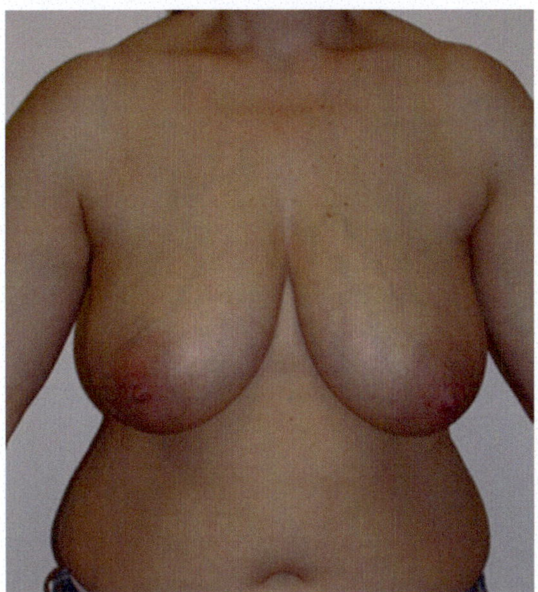

Fig. 5.35

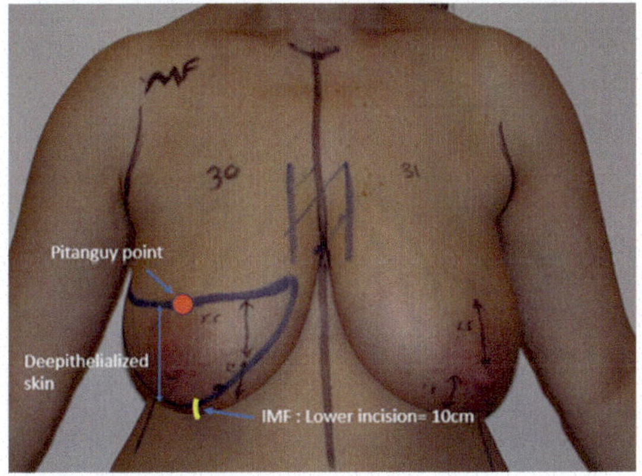

Fig. 5.36

ing capsule or capsular flaps as outlined above in our algorithm for lateral and inferior malposition [9, 10].

Case Analysis

The patient is a 67-year-old female who presented with post reconstruction deformity including misshapen breasts and symmastia. She originally underwent bilateral nipple-sparing mastectomies and direct-to-implant technique in the subpectoral pocket using tear-shaped 310-cc (with x, y, z of 12/11/5.2 cm) gel implants and ADM at a different institution. She developed symmastia and shape asymmetry. Her surgeon tried revising it by operating on the right side only. He performed medial pocket reconstruction with capsular flap and reinforcement with Seri Surgical Scaffold and used a 350-cc tear-shaped implant to add more projection to the right side.

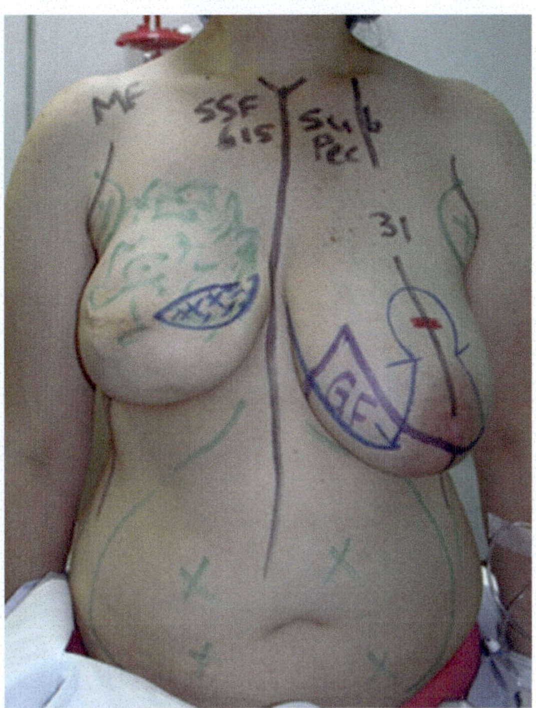

Fig. 5.37

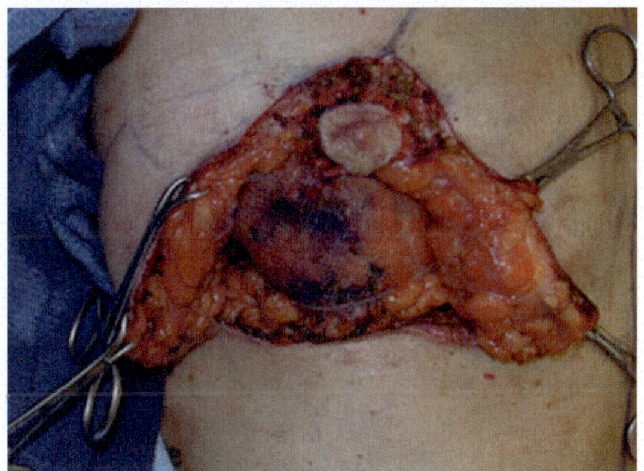

Fig. 5.38

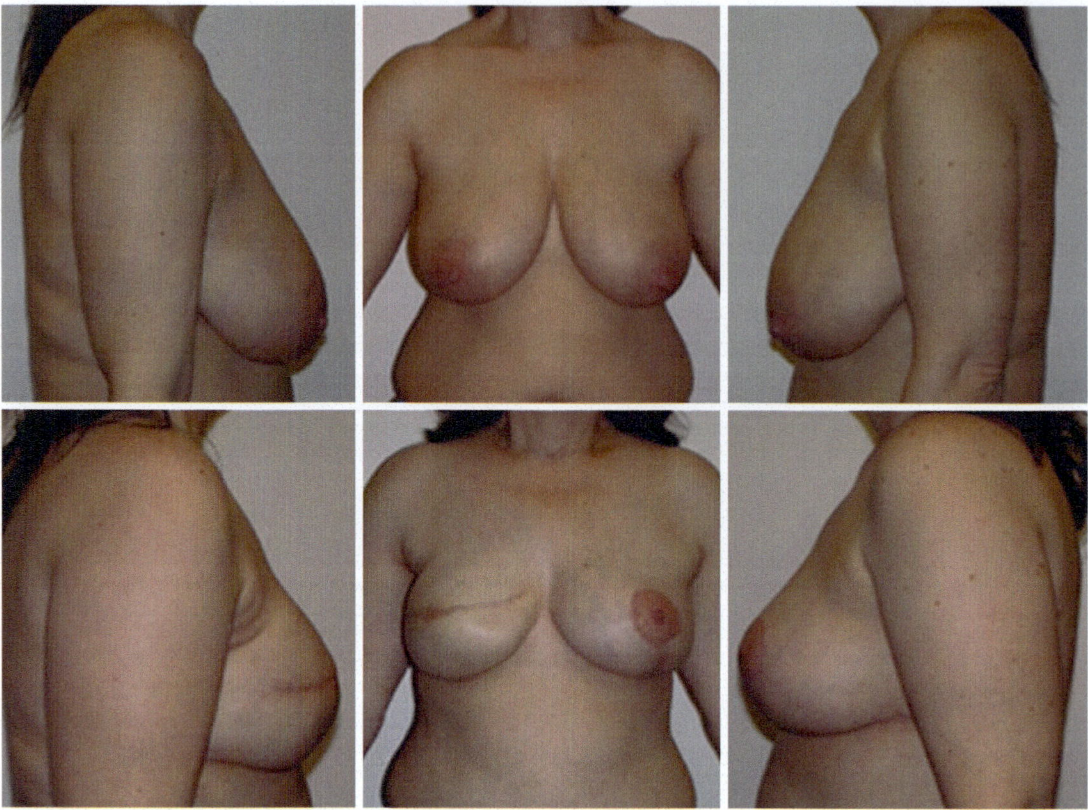

Fig. 5.39

She subsequently redeveloped the same problem and sought a second opinion.

On examination, she had grossly misshapen breasts with contracted envelope inferolaterally, symmastia, severe pectus excavatum with different levels of chest AP projection, and, hence, different levels of implant projection. In addition, she had animation deformity and paucity of subcutaneous tissue with visible rippling (Fig. 5.40).

Treatment-wise, she did not want to have autologous flap reconstruction due to its morbidity. We strategically planned on having a fresh start given the previous failures in the subpectoral pockets, presence of the Seri mesh, severe pectus excavatum, and contracted envelope inferolaterally. We planned to perform a two-stage reconstruction, with the first stage aimed at bilateral partial capsulectomies laterally, change of pockets to prepectoral space, and limiting the medial pocket dissection given the unfavorable downward slope of the ribs medially (Fig. 5.41).

During the surgery, the level of complexity of her chest pectus excavatum anatomy became even more evident (Fig. 5.42).

During the ensuing expansion, the skin envelope expanded favorably. After 6 months, she underwent the second stage with 450-cc tear-shaped implants (13/13.5/6.1 cm) and fat injection to the sternum, upper chest, and breasts (140 cc on the right side and 90 cc on the left side) (Fig. 5.43). It was felt that given her level of chest asymmetry, the best option was to use the same implants on both sides and try to improve the contour symmetry with fat injection.

Postoperatively, she had much improved cosmesis with better breast shape and symmetry with correction of symmastia (Fig. 5.44). She, however, continues to have rippling and implant visibility that can benefit from more fat injection. Perhaps, addition of ADM at the time of her stage I surgery or in the future may help in improving this issue.

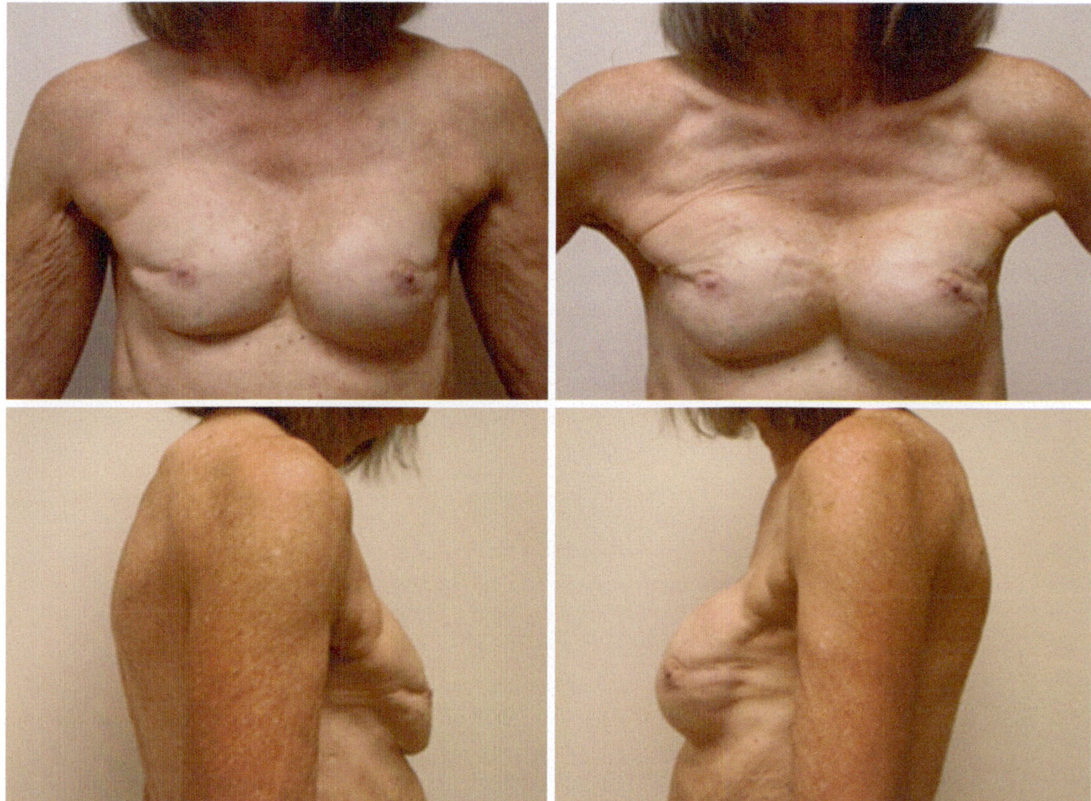

Fig. 5.40

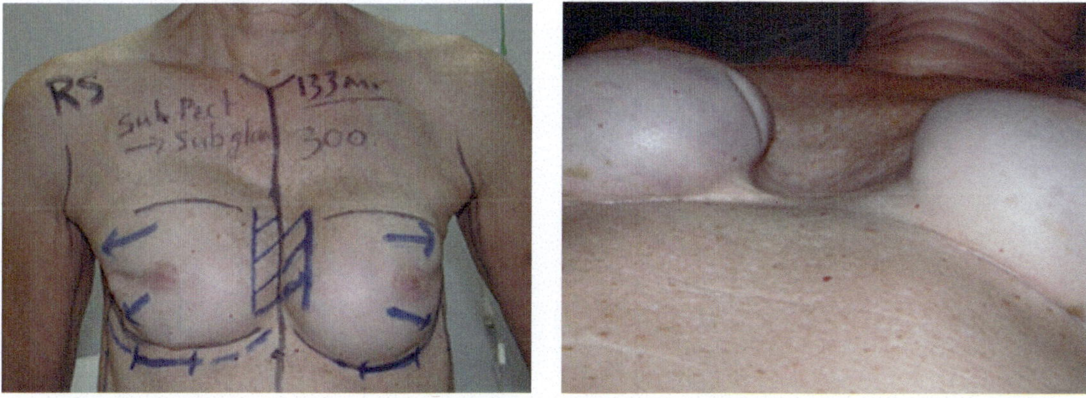

Fig. 5.41

Fig. 5.42

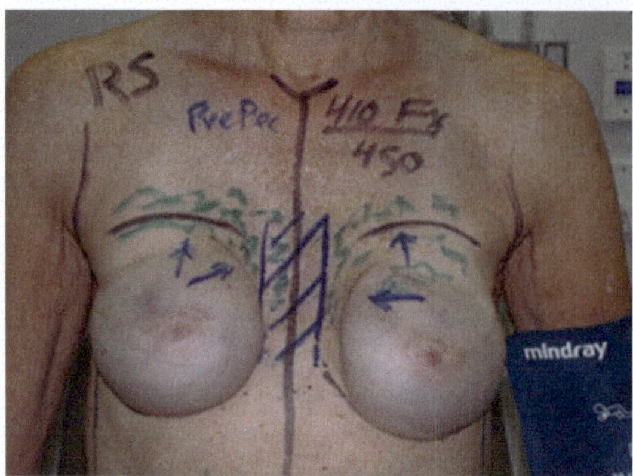

Fig. 5.43

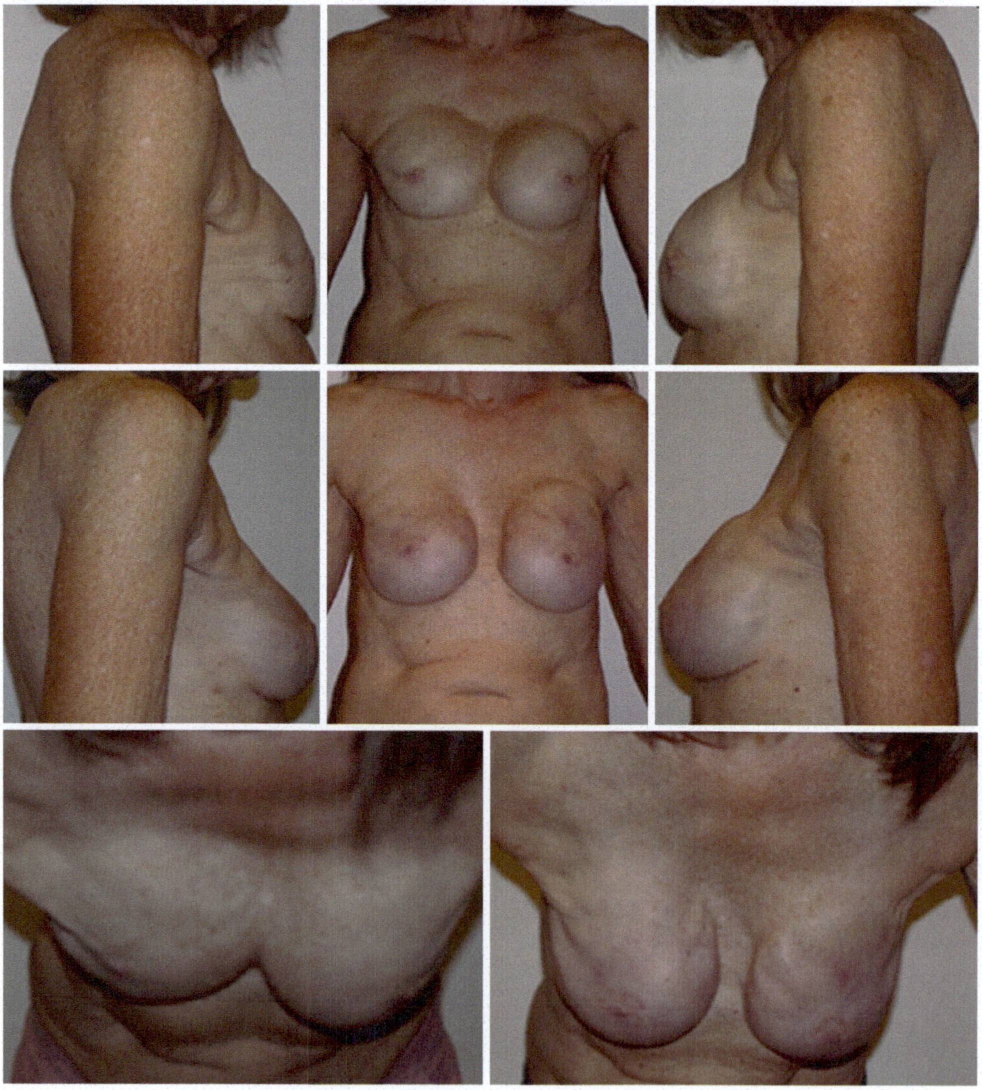

Fig. 5.44

Conclusion

This chapter reviews and demonstrates management of some of the most challenging cases that we face in our practices. The best practice principles that we have discussed in the previous four chapters are still the compass that we need to use to not only to avoid complications but also to help with revision surgery. One must also remember that sometimes the best treatment is to have a fresh start in revision breast surgery.

References

1. Dickinson BP, Handel N. Approaching revisional surgery in augmentation and mastopexy/augmentation patients. Ann Plast Surg. 2012;68:12–6.
2. Suri S, Bagiella E, Factor S, Taub P. Soft tissue adjuncts in revisionary breast revisionary aesthetic surgery. Ann Plast Surg. 2107;78:230–5.
3. Brown MH, Somogyi RB, Aggarwal S. Secondary breast augmentation. Plast Reconstr Surg. 2016;138:119e.
4. Patrick Maxwell G, Gabriel A. Acellular dermal matrix for reoperative breast augmentation. Plast Reconstr Surg. 2014;134:932.
5. Moskovitz MJ, Baxt SA, Jain AK, Hausman RE. Liposuction breast reduction: a prospective trial in African American women. Plast Reconstr Surg. 2007;119:718.
6. Shultz K, Movassaghi K. Correction of implant malposition. Presented at ASAPS meeting in New York, 2018. Best paper award.
7. Spear SL, Seruya M, Clemens MW, Teitelbaum S, Nahabedian MY. Acellular dermal matrix for the treatment and prevention of implant-associated breast deformities. Plast Reconstr Surg. 2011;127:1047.
8. Adams WP Jr, Baxter R, Glicksman C, Mast BA, Tantillo M, Van Natta BW. The use of poly-4-hydroxybutyrate (P4HB) scaffold in the ptotic breast: a multicenter clinical study. Aesthet Surg J. 2018;38(5):502–18.
9. Spear SL, Dayan JH, Bogue D, Clemens MW, Newman M, Teitelbaum S, et al. The "neosubpectoral" pocket for the correction of symmastia. Plast Reconstr Surg. 2009;124:695.
10. Parsa FD. Breast capsulopexy for capsular ptosis after augmentation mammoplasty. Plast Reconstr Surg. 1990;85(5):809–12.

Index

K. Movassaghi (ed.), *Shaping the Breast*, https://doi.org/10.1007/978-3-030-59777-1

The manufacturer's authorised representative in the EU is Springer Nature Customer Service Centre GmbH, Europaplatz 3, 69115 Heidelberg, Germany. If you have any concerns regarding our products, please contact ProductSafety@springernature.com

Printed and bound by CPI Group (UK) Ltd, Croydon, CR0 4YY
15/07/2026
02167655-0003